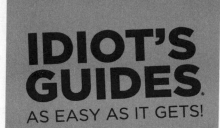

IDIOT'S GUIDES.

AS EASY AS IT GETS!

Overcoming Type 2 Diabetes

by Carrie S. Swift, MS, RDN, CDE, with Nathaniel G. Clark, MD, MS, RD

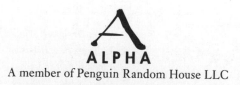

ALPHA

A member of Penguin Random House LLC

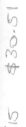

JB   07/15 $30.51

This book is dedicated to all people who courageously live with diabetes.

ALPHA BOOKS

Published by Penguin Random House LLC

Penguin Random House LLC, 375 Hudson Street, New York, New York 10014, USA • Penguin Random House LLC (Canada), 90 Eglinton Avenue East, Suite 700, Toronto, Ontario M4P 2Y3, Canada (a division of Pearson Penguin Canada Inc.) • Penguin Books Ltd., 80 Strand, London WC2R 0RL, England • Penguin Ireland, 25 St. Stephen's Green, Dublin 2, Ireland (a division of Penguin Books Ltd.) • Penguin Random House LLC (Australia), 250 Camberwell Road, Camberwell, Victoria 3124, Australia (a division of Pearson Australia Group Pty. Ltd.) • Penguin Books India Pvt. Ltd., 11 Community Centre, Panchsheel Park, New Delhi—110 017, India • Penguin Random House LLC (NZ), 67 Apollo Drive, Rosedale, North Shore, Auckland 1311, New Zealand (a division of Pearson New Zealand Ltd.) • Penguin Books (South Africa) (Pty.) Ltd., 24 Sturdee Avenue, Rosebank, Johannesburg 2196, South Africa • Penguin Books Ltd., Registered Offices: 80 Strand, London WC2R 0RL, England

001-278656-July2015

International Standard Book Number: 978-1-61564-792-7
Library of Congress Catalog Card Number: 2014959610

17 16 15   8 7 6 5 4 3 2 1

Interpretation of the printing code: The rightmost number of the first series of numbers is the year of the book's printing; the rightmost number of the second series of numbers is the number of the book's printing. For example, a printing code of 15-1 shows that the first printing occurred in 2015.

Printed in the United States of America

Note: This publication contains the opinions and ideas of its authors. It is intended to provide helpful and informative material on the subject matter covered. It is sold with the understanding that the authors and publisher are not engaged in rendering professional services in the book. If the reader requires personal assistance or advice, a competent professional should be consulted. The authors and publisher specifically disclaim any responsibility for any liability, loss, or risk, personal or otherwise, which is incurred as a consequence, directly or indirectly, of the use and application of any of the contents of this book.

Most Alpha books are available at special quantity discounts for bulk purchases for sales promotions, premiums, fundraising, or educational use. Special books, or book excerpts, can also be created to fit specific needs. For details, write: Special Markets, Alpha Books, 375 Hudson Street, New York, NY 10014.

Publisher: *Mike Sanders*
Associate Publisher: *Billy Fields*
Acquisitions Editor: *Janette Lynn*
Development Editor: *Kayla Dugger*
Cover Designer: *Laura Merriman*

Book Designer: *William Thomas*
Indexer: *Brad Herriman*
Layout: *Ayanna Lacey*
Proofreader: *Laura Caddell*

Contents

Appenidixes

Introduction

More people than ever before have diabetes. According to the Centers for Disease Control and Prevention (CDC), there are 29.1 million Americans with diabetes—almost double the population of New York City, Los Angeles, and Chicago combined. Of the 9.3 percent of people living in the United States that have diabetes, the large majority (95 percent) have type 2 diabetes. And $176 billion—yes, that's with a *b*—was spent on direct diabetes medical costs in 2012 alone. These statistics illustrate the scope of the problem. Diabetes is something that needs to be taken seriously.

However, because diabetes is big business, many want to throw their hat in the ring to get in on it. As a result, much of the material you come across is not always accurate or helpful. Sometimes you see scams designed to take your money or encouraging you to buy products you don't need. Other times, information you access can actually be harmful if acted upon. And when you do find something valid, it isn't always easy to understand—it might be too clinical or feel like data overload. That's where *Idiot's Guides: Overcoming Type 2 Diabetes* comes in.

From a primer on diabetes medications and their side effects to how different foods can affect your health, this book not only teaches you how to effectively manage your diabetes, but also how to live your life with success and satisfaction while doing so. After all, you just happen to be a person who has diabetes; it is not who you are as a person. With this book, we're aiming to help you overcome diabetes so it doesn't overcome you!

How This Book Is Organized

The material in this book is presented in six parts so you can easily find what you're looking for on the subject of diabetes.

Part 1, Defining Diabetes, reviews what type 2 diabetes is, as well as the other forms of diabetes. We also bust some common myths about diabetes and show you where you can find the most accurate resources on the internet.

Part 2, Putting Yourself on the Right Path, starts off with how to make positive behavior changes, including identifying a meaningful change that you want to make, setting goals, and measuring your success. Because support for your diabetes management efforts is critical to success, we also walk you through who you need on your diabetes care team and how to ask for support from family and friends. We close this part with information on how to avoid short- and long-term complications associated with diabetes, as well as how others can help you with this.

Part 3, Diabetes Management Strategies, addresses ways to manage your diabetes. We start by talking about upping your physical activity, even if it's just adding a few more steps to your day. Insulin and various diabetes medications are also reviewed in this part, with clear explanations of how the medications work and what's new. We then explain how insulin pumps and glucose sensors work, and how to use blood glucose meters. What action to take based on your blood glucose results is also revealed in this part. Finally, we discuss different changes you can make to better control your blood glucose, from managing stress to getting a good night's sleep.

Part 4, Food as Medicine, provides an in-depth nutrition review on what foods can help and hurt you health wise. You get information on how food affects your blood glucose, as well as how to decrease the ones that aren't good for it. We also include healthy eating strategies and information on how to read food labels.

Part 5, Diabetes Meal Planning, reviews the glycemic index and four evidence-based diabetes eating plans and provides sample one-day menus for each. Weight-loss strategies and secrets to success are also included in this part. We conclude with tips on how to gauge your progress.

Part 6, Special Considerations: Older Adults and Families, discusses unique aspects of diabetes management in older adults, including nutrition needs, physical activity, and medications. Lifestyle tips for families affected by diabetes are also shared to help prevent and manage type 2 diabetes in children.

Extras

Throughout the book, you will notice sidebars providing four types of information about diabetes.

 DEFINITION

Definitions are included to ensure the text is easy to understand, without distractions from complex medical terms or unfamiliar words related to diabetes.

 DIABETES DECODED

You'll find diabetes "insider information" and tips you can use in these sidebars. If there's something extra to help you manage your diabetes, it will be shared here.

 DID YOU KNOW?

These sidebars provide facts or supplemental material you might find interesting. This is where you can learn just a little more about specific diabetes topics in the main text.

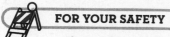 **FOR YOUR SAFETY**

> These sidebars call your attention to important safety messages you don't want to miss. Topics like medication side effects or things known to worsen diabetes control will be highlighted here.

Acknowledgments

I'd like to thank Janette Lynn and the team at Alpha Books for giving me the opportunity to author this book.

I'd also like to thank Nathaniel Clark, MD, MS, RD, who generously gave of his time to provide the technical review. I appreciate his insight, knowledge, and expertise. I was delighted to get to collaborate with him on this project.

Thank you to my diabetes colleagues, friends, and family who have always encouraged me to step outside of my comfort zone and take on new things. And to my clients, friends, and family living with diabetes who inspired me to write this book, I have learned so much from all of you.

Most importantly, thank you to my wonderful family, my husband Neil, and our daughter Erin. I greatly appreciate their love, support, and patience during the writing of this book.

—Carrie S. Swift, MS, RDN, BC-ADM, CDE

Special Thanks to the Technical Reviewer

Idiot's Guides: Overcoming Type 2 Diabetes was reviewed by a content expert who double-checked the accuracy of what you'll learn here, to help us ensure this book gives you everything you need to know about diabetes. Special thanks are extended to Nathaniel G. Clark, MD, MS, RD.

Trademarks

All terms mentioned in this book that are known to be or are suspected of being trademarks or service marks have been appropriately capitalized. Alpha Books and Penguin Random House LLC cannot attest to the accuracy of this information. Use of a term in this book should not be regarded as affecting the validity of any trademark or service mark.

Defining Diabetes

Before you jump into how to treat type 2 diabetes, you first need to know more about what diabetes is. So in this part, we give you a primer on type 2 diabetes, as well as other types of diabetes. Through this, you'll gain understanding of what causes diabetes, who gets it, and how you know for sure if you have it.

We then help you separate myth from fact when it comes to diabetes, with tips on how to identify the useful information to develop your diabetes self-management skills.

What Is Type 2 Diabetes?

If you just found out that you, a friend, or a member of your family has type 2 diabetes, you are not alone. The number of people around the world with type 2 diabetes is growing at a rapid pace. You probably have quite a few questions about the seriousness of this diagnosis and what to do about it.

In this chapter, we help you understand what type 2 diabetes is, who gets it, and how it is diagnosed.

In This Chapter

- Defining type 2 diabetes
- Risk factors for type 2 diabetes
- What are the symptoms?
- Diagnosing type 2 diabetes

Not the Serious Kind of Diabetes?

While many people have heard that type 2 diabetes isn't as serious as type 1 diabetes, it is actually a complex, chronic condition that those in the medical field continue to learn new information about all the time.

Your body metabolizes, or breaks down, much of the food you eat into glucose—a type of sugar. Insulin is needed to get the glucose from your blood into your cells, where it is used for energy or stored for later use. With type 2 diabetes, your body is generally not using insulin well; this is called *insulin resistance.* Eventually, not enough insulin can be made to overcome the resistance and the glucose builds up in your blood, leading to high blood glucose or "blood sugar," medically known as hyperglycemia (see Chapter 6 for more on hyperglycemia).

> **DID YOU KNOW?**
>
> Insulin is made by the beta cells of the pancreas. When the pancreas is working normally, insulin is released into the blood at the right time in the right amounts when glucose goes up, like after a meal. Insulin not only helps glucose get into your cells, it also helps your body store fat.

However, type 2 is not "just a touch of sugar." It can lead to problems with your heart, eyes, kidneys, and blood vessels and cause nerve damage if your blood glucose remains elevated. Sometimes there are additional risk factors—for instance, you may have a family history of heart disease in addition to diabetes—and multiple factors can make it more likely for a problem to develop.

How Type 2 Diabetes Develops

Though there really is no such thing as *borderline diabetes,* the term is still commonly used. Having borderline diabetes is like being borderline pregnant! You may start out with normal blood glucose, develop prediabetes, and then progress to type 2 diabetes. But once you have diabetes, you have diabetes. The following image shows the basic progression to type 2 based on insulin resistance, blood glucose, and insulin production.

No diabetes: Generally insulin resistance starts early, even before diabetes is diagnosed. The body is basically ignoring the insulin, so the cells think they are starving. The message is sent out to release stored sugar and the blood glucose starts to go higher. The beta cells in the pancreas go into overdrive, making more insulin to keep up with the higher amount of glucose in the blood.

Prediabetes: The blood glucose starts to gradually rise due to the insulin resistance and as the beta cells start lagging behind in insulin production.

Type 2 diabetes: Over time, the beta cells continue lagging farther behind and eventually can't keep up. Those cells start to burn out, so to speak. Once that happens, the blood glucose is in the diabetes range.

How Type 2 Diabetes Progresses

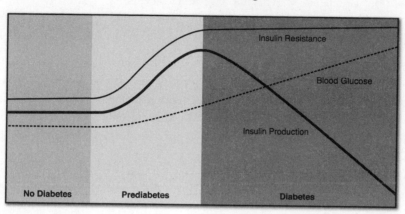

The time that this takes to happen varies from person to person. Sometimes diabetes can be managed with meal planning and physical activity for quite a while; for others, diabetes medications are needed right away; and still others need insulin from the time they are diagnosed, potentially only for a short time. But due to the progressive nature of type 2 diabetes, what may manage your diabetes today may not work as well in the future.

At some point in time, you may need insulin. If you do need insulin to manage your blood glucose, it means you have a beta cell failure; you have an exhausted pancreas that no longer produces enough insulin. You therefore need to replace the insulin you used to make with insulin that you take. Taking insulin doesn't mean you have a worse type of diabetes or that type 2 diabetes turns into type 1 diabetes. It is simply used to keep blood glucose on target.

Who Gets Type 2?

In the past, type 2 diabetes was referred to as *adult-onset diabetes* or *non-insulin-dependent diabetes*. However, each of these terms is inaccurate when it comes to people who get type 2 diabetes.

Unfortunately, over the past 20 years, children and teenagers have also been developing type 2 diabetes with increasing frequency. This is, at least in part, due to higher rates of obesity and inactivity in children and teens. According to the Centers for Disease Control and Prevention (CDC), type 2 diabetes in youth is generally diagnosed in obese children and teens between the ages of 10 and 19 years who have a strong family history of type 2 diabetes. It is no longer a problem just for adults.

And while most people with type 2 diabetes are still *making* insulin, *taking* insulin may still be needed to reach your blood glucose targets. The CDC identifies approximately 29 percent of people with diabetes in the United States who take insulin alone or in combination with other diabetes medications to control their blood glucose. Because people with type 2 diabetes make up 90 to 95 percent of the population with diabetes, we know that insulin is not used just in the treatment of type 1 diabetes (see Chapter 2 for more on type 1). Still, many people—even some health-care providers—still think that once a person starts taking insulin, that person has type 1 diabetes. This isn't the case; insulin is simply another tool to achieve improved blood glucose control. It does not change the type of diabetes you have.

So as you can see, adults and people who don't need insulin aren't the only ones at risk for type 2 diabetes; people across all age ranges and health needs in the general population are at risk, too. In fact, according to the CDC, there are a full 86 million people who have prediabetes and are at high risk of developing type 2 diabetes, as well as approximately 27.5 million with type 2 diabetes in the United States. It seems almost everyone in the United States either has, loves someone who has, or knows someone who has diabetes.

Risk Factors

What are the risk factors for developing type 2 diabetes? Certain groups have a higher risk, including Hispanics/Latinos, Asian Americans, African Americans, Pacific Islanders, and American Indians.

 DIABETES DECODED

The same strategies used in the Diabetes Prevention Program (DPP) are useful in managing type 2 diabetes. It doesn't take losing a large amount of weight to see a big improvement in blood glucose. Aim to lose 7 percent of your body weight. To calculate the amount, take your weight in pounds and multiply by .07. For example: 190 × .07 = 13.3. So the target weight loss would be 13 pounds. One of the best ways to start increasing your activity is walking. Moderate activity of 150 minutes a week may not be easy to work into your schedule, but it is okay to break it down to 10 minutes at a time. Can you fit in 10 more minutes of activity somewhere in your day? Start with that and work your way up to 150 minutes a week. You can do it! (See Chapter 7 for more on how to get moving.)

The following are additional risk factors for type 2 diabetes:

- A family history of diabetes

- Being over 45 years old

- Being overweight—if you store extra fat in your middle, you have a higher risk than if you store extra fat in your hips and thighs

- Physical inactivity

- For women, if you gave birth to a baby weighing more than 9 pounds or had gestational diabetes during pregnancy

- Prediabetes or polycystic ovary syndrome (PCOS)

However, just because you may have risk factors for type 2 diabetes doesn't mean it is inevitable that you will get it. A large clinical research study called the Diabetes Prevention Program (DPP) was conducted at multiple centers across the United States on overweight people with prediabetes to discover if losing a modest amount of weight by changing eating habits and increasing physical activity or treatment with the diabetes medication metformin would delay or prevent type 2 diabetes. Participants who lost weight by increasing activity and making healthy changes to their eating habits had a significant decrease in the risk of developing diabetes, something shown to be particularly beneficial to those age 60 and older. Meanwhile, participants taking metformin reduced their diabetes risk by 31 percent, which particularly benefitted people ages 25 to 44 years old and at least 60 pounds overweight. So the DPP results tell us that eating healthier and moving more really do make a difference in prevention.

How Genetics and Environment Play a Role

While it's true there are definitely things you can do to decrease your risk of developing type 2 diabetes, you could do everything possible and still end up with diabetes. And the opposite is true as well—there are a number of people who are overweight and inactive who don't have diabetes, and probably never will. This could be due to genetics. In fact, there is a strong genetic link for type 2 diabetes, but it isn't always predictable who will get it.

Environmental factors are also a trigger. Type 2 diabetes is common in families not only due to the genetics, but also due to the home environment. For example, children in a family may be overweight and inactive because the parents are, too. But families that center their time around activity and exercise rather than eating high-calorie snack foods while watching TV are less likely to develop diabetes even when they have the same genetic risks.

Is your diabetes a result of your genes? Was it triggered by lifestyle factors? The answer is usually "yes" to both questions. While you can't change your genetics or your family history, you can change your environment and make healthier lifestyle choices, as you'll learn about more in this book.

> **DID YOU KNOW?**
>
> The International Diabetes Federation (IDF) estimates that 382 million people across the globe are living with diabetes. Similar to the United States, at least 90 percent of people with diabetes have type 2 diabetes. And while the percentage of the population with diabetes is larger in the United States, the sheer number of people with diabetes in countries like China (98 million) and India (65 million) is actually much higher and on the rise. Why is this happening in China and India? The genetic predisposition for type 2 diabetes is more common in these populations. This is due to the "westernization" of these countries when it comes to food (fast food and other convenience food choices) and a lower rate of physical activity in overcrowded cities with poor air quality. These issues lead to an increase in environmental triggers for the already present genetic risk.

How Do You Know You Have It?

If you are an adult age 45 and older, or are an overweight younger adult with one additional diabetes risk factor, you should complete a blood glucose screening. A routine screening at the doctor's office is often what leads to a diagnosis. If you don't fall into either of those categories, you should still learn about the symptoms. Catching diabetes early and managing it well will help contribute to long-term success.

Symptoms—Why You May Not Have Noticed

You may have had diabetes for years without knowing it. The reason for this is that not everyone has symptoms or that the change is so gradual it goes unnoticed. Diabetes symptoms include the following:

- **Increased thirst:** This occurs when the extra glucose in the blood is drawing fluid from your body tissues, which causes you to drink more. You could guzzle down liquids all day long and still feel thirsty, because you are not able to get hydrated.

- **Frequent urination (having to pee a lot):** Because you are drinking more due to the fluid being drawn from your tissues, you may need to urinate more.

- **Increased hunger:** When you don't have enough insulin to get glucose from your blood into your cells, your body reacts by releasing stored glucose and making additional glucose. Eventually the stored glucose from the muscles and organs is used up, triggering extreme hunger. You could eat all day and still be starving.

- **Fatigue (being tired all the time):** When your cells can't get the energy they need and your stored sugar is used up, you may feel tired and probably more than a bit cranky.

- **Weight loss without trying to lose weight:** When blood sugars are high, glucose spills out into the urine. This means you are actually urinating out calories. Your body then tries to adapt by using stored fat and protein as energy sources to substitute for the glucose it's not able to use, which can cause the loss of lean muscle mass along with fat.

- **Blurry vision:** With high blood sugar, the lenses of your eyes can swell, making it more difficult to see. This is usually temporary and stabilizes once your blood sugar improves.

- **Slow-healing cuts and wounds:** Elevated blood glucose leads to stiffened, narrow arteries, which in turn contribute to poor circulation. This lowers the blood flow of nutrients and oxygen to a wound, which slows the healing process.

- **Frequent infections—for example, women getting urinary tract and/or yeast infections:** The immune system is also affected by high blood sugars, making it harder for your body to fight off infections.

 DID YOU KNOW?

The American Diabetes Association (ADA) offers a free one-minute diabetes risk test that determines your risk level for developing type 2 diabetes at diabetes.org/are-you-at-risk. If you have diabetes, members of your family may also be at risk. Encourage them to take the risk test and be screened if it is recommended.

Diagnosing Type 2 Diabetes

Type 2 diabetes is diagnosed by a fasting blood glucose test or an A1C test done at a lab, which your medical provider will order for you (see Chapter 11 for more on A1C). Because the blood glucose test is done fasting, it is usually done in the morning. An A1C test, which does not require fasting, is a blood test that measures average blood glucose for the past two to three months and is reported as a percentage value. To complete either test, you go to a lab and have a blood sample drawn from your arm. The blood is then processed by the lab to get the result. Though not usually for an initial diagnosis, an A1C test may alternatively be run on a machine at your medical provider's office from a finger-stick blood sample. Results are generally available within a few minutes when that method of testing is used. In most cases, one fasting blood glucose and/or A1C test is enough to diagnose diabetes. However, if the test results don't clearly indicate diabetes, they are usually repeated on another day to confirm the diagnosis.

In some cases, an oral glucose tolerance test (OGTT) may also be performed to diagnose diabetes. An OGTT measures blood glucose before and after drinking a sugary liquid containing a specific amount of glucose (usually 75 grams [g]). Blood is drawn from your arm at 30 minutes, 60 minutes, and then again at 2 hours. If the blood glucose goes up and remains elevated during this test, it may indicate diabetes. The two-hour blood glucose result is the one that is used to diagnose type 2 diabetes.

So what numbers are indicative of type 2 diabetes? The following table lists the results that would lead to a diagnosis of type 2 diabetes. Some of the results are presented in milligrams per deciliter (mg/dL), which indicates the concentration of blood glucose.

Test Numbers That Indicate Type 2 Diabetes

Test	Result to Diagnose Diabetes
Fasting blood glucose (eight or more hours since eating)	≥126 mg/dL
Random blood glucose with hyperglycemia symptoms	≥200 mg/dL
A1C	≥6.5%
Two-hour blood glucose during an OGTT	≥200 mg/dL

Source: Diagnostic Criteria—American Diabetes Association 2014

DIABETES DECODED

Some people think eating more sweets or drinking more sugary soft drinks before being tested for diabetes can give a false result. Unfortunately, that's not the case. When everything is functioning normally, the pancreas works to keep the blood glucose balanced no matter what foods are eaten. So the results you receive are not a "false positive" based on what you ate in the days or even weeks leading up to a blood glucose test indicating diabetes.

If you have been diagnosed with diabetes, the important thing is to achieve better blood glucose management now that you know what you're dealing with.

Is There a Cure?

Right now, there is no cure for diabetes. However, treatment options are developing quickly as type 2 diabetes is better understood. New diabetes medications are constantly in development that approach diabetes control in different ways (see Chapter 11 for more on diabetes medications), and healthy eating and physical activity make up the foundation for the treatment of type 2 diabetes. This enhanced understanding of diabetes may help lead to an eventual cure.

Plus, new prevention strategies are also being explored. There is evidence that demonstrates getting blood glucose closer to normal early on has long-lasting benefits in preventing complications of diabetes. This has led to measures aimed at improving the quality of diabetes care and how it is managed in the United States. An example of how the evidence has shaped diabetes treatment is that diabetes pills are being used more frequently right at the time of diagnosis.

So don't be afraid to talk to your doctor to see what you need to do to improve control of your blood glucose. It may be one of the best things you can do. You don't want to wait until you feel bad to take action.

 FOR YOUR SAFETY

If you were prescribed diabetes medication(s), make sure you know the possible side effects and how it works. Ask your prescribing provider, the pharmacist where you fill your prescriptions, or a diabetes educator to review this information with you. If there are medications you take that you don't understand why you are taking them, ask the prescribing provider. You should always know why you are taking a medication and the expected benefits, along with potential side effects.

The Least You Need to Know

- Type 2 diabetes is a serious chronic condition that can be well managed.
- According to the CDC, 86 million people in the United States have prediabetes and are at high risk of developing type 2 diabetes.
- Type 2 diabetes is diagnosed via a fasting blood glucose, A1C, or OGTT test.
- Healthy eating habits and physical activity are the cornerstones of treating diabetes. Diabetes medication or insulin may also be needed to treat type 2 diabetes.

Other Types of Diabetes

Although much of this book focuses on managing type 2 diabetes, it helps to understand other types of diabetes, as diabetes care strategies often overlap. So in this chapter, we discuss the most common types of diabetes aside from type 2—including type 1 and gestational diabetes—as well as the less-common types and causes.

In This Chapter

- Defining type 1 diabetes
- Differences between type 1 and type 2 diabetes
- Gestational diabetes
- Lesser-known types of diabetes
- Diabetes caused by pancreatitis, cystic fibrosis, and chemicals and medications

Type 1 Diabetes

Type 1 diabetes used to be referred to as juvenile-onset diabetes because it is generally diagnosed in children, teens, and young adults. Even though type 1 diabetes is typically diagnosed in youth, it can potentially show up at any age. Unlike type 2 diabetes, which comes on gradually, type 1 diabetes appears suddenly, without warning. Five percent of people with diabetes have type 1 diabetes. The following are some current facts about type 1 diabetes according to the JDRF (formerly known as the Juvenile Diabetes Research Foundation):

- Approximately 3 million Americans have type 1 diabetes.

- An estimated 15,000 adults and 15,000 children are diagnosed annually in the United States—80 people a day.

- Nearly 85 percent of people in the United States with type 1 diabetes are adults; 15 percent are children.

- The number of cases of type 1 diabetes in the United States in those under age 20 went up 23 percent from 2001 to 2009.

- Worldwide, the number of children diagnosed with type 1 diabetes is expected to rise 3 percent each year.

As regards younger people diagnosed with type 1, it is true that the longer you live with diabetes, the more likely complications may occur. So for someone who is very young at diagnosis, they will be living many more years with diabetes, and complications are more likely to happen over their lifetime.

What Causes Type 1 Diabetes?

Type 1 diabetes is an *autoimmune disease* that occurs when the body's own immune system attacks and destroys the beta cells of the pancreas that make insulin. When insulin is not produced, glucose builds up in the blood and can quickly lead to serious consequences. People with type 1 diabetes must take insulin to live; multiple daily injections and insulin pumps (more on this later in Chapter 10) are frequently used to manage type 1 diabetes.

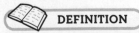 **DEFINITION**

Autoimmune disease occurs when the body's tissues are assaulted by their own immune system. The immune system is designed to seek out and destroy invaders of the body to provide protection from bacteria, viruses, and cancer. Damage is caused when the immune system becomes misdirected and attacks the body tissues it is designed to protect. **Autoantibodies** are proteins produced by the immune system that react to its own cells and tissues in autoimmune disease.

It is not fully known why the body attacks the beta cells of the pancreas, leading to type 1 diabetes. But in many people, the stage may actually be set years before it appears. Researchers have found that relatives of people with type 1 diabetes who later developed diabetes had *autoantibodies* in their blood for years prior to being diagnosed.

Symptoms of type 1 diabetes can happen quickly and may include the following:

- Extreme thirst and dry mouth

- Being tired or drowsy

- Sudden weight loss

- Frequent urination

- Sudden changes in vision

- Difficulty breathing

- Confusion

- Fruity odor to the breath

- Stomach pain, nausea, or vomiting

- Loss of consciousness

While these symptoms may be the first sign of type 1 diabetes, they can also happen anytime blood glucose is very high. These warning signs could even indicate *diabetic ketoacidosis (DKA)*. If you or anyone you know has symptoms of DKA, seek immediate medical attention. If someone is experiencing difficulty breathing or loss of consciousness, call 911 right away. Emergency medical treatment is also needed if stomach pain, nausea, and vomiting are combined with any of the other symptoms from the list of type 1 diabetes symptoms.

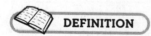 **DEFINITION**

Diabetic ketoacidosis (DKA) is a life-threatening condition that affects people with diabetes, especially type 1 diabetes. It happens when there is not enough insulin for the body to use the glucose in the blood as fuel; instead, fat becomes the fuel source. As fat is broken down, ketones are produced as a waste product. High levels of ketones in the blood become toxic and can be caused by missed or inadequate insulin doses in conditions such as infection, surgery, or injury.

Differences from Type 2

When people hear the word *diabetes,* they generally think about type 2 diabetes, especially when thinking about prevention strategies and weight management. Unfortunately, it isn't possible to prevent type 1 diabetes at this time. While both types of diabetes are associated with environmental triggers and genetic predisposition, lifestyle factors have nothing to do with the onset of type 1 diabetes; it can't be prevented by eating healthy and exercising.

Whereas type 2 diabetes runs in families, that's not the case with type 1 diabetes. If someone has type 1 diabetes, it is much less likely that immediate family members also have type 1 diabetes. In fact, only about 15 percent of people with type 1 diabetes have first-degree relatives who have it, too. Usually for type 1 diabetes to occur, risk factors must be inherited from both parents. It is believed that these risk factors are more common among whites, because there is a higher incidence of type 1 diabetes in whites. The good news is that the majority of people who inherit the risk factors never go on to develop the disease. That's why environmental triggers are suspected.

Type 1 diabetes is more common in colder climates and is diagnosed more often in the winter than in the summer. For example, countries with a high incidence of type 1 diabetes in children include Finland and Sweden. In contrast, incidence of type 2 diabetes is unrelated to climate or time of year. Viruses are another potential trigger for type 1 diabetes. The same virus that might be a nuisance for many people may be the final straw that triggers type 1 diabetes in others. Type 1 diabetes also appears to be less common in people who were breastfed as infants and had solid foods introduced later when they were babies.

While the blood glucose and A1C criteria to diagnose type 1 diabetes are the same as type 2, several additional blood tests—though not required to make the diagnosis—may be ordered. Sometimes it is difficult to clearly identify what type of diabetes the person has. Generally these tests would be ordered to confirm a diagnosis of type 1 diabetes when type 2 diabetes has not yet been ruled out. As a by-product of insulin production, c-peptide is ordered to determine the level of insulin still being produced. Because little to no insulin is made with type 1 diabetes, an abnormally low level of c-peptide would be expected with the diagnosis of type 1 diabetes, unlike with type 2.

 DID YOU KNOW?

While genetic predisposition is common to both type 1 diabetes and type 2 diabetes, there is a stronger genetic link for type 2. Studies of identical twins have provided insight as to genetic predisposition. When an identical twin has type 1 diabetes, there is about a 50-50 chance of the other twin getting it. On the other hand, with type 2 diabetes, there is an approximate three out of four likelihood the second identical twin will develop the disease.

Gestational Diabetes

Gestational diabetes is glucose intolerance that is first recognized or begins during pregnancy. During pregnancy, the amount of insulin needed to control blood glucose goes up. Hormones that help support the growth of the baby also decrease the action of the mom's insulin. The mother may need up to three times more insulin than before pregnancy just to keep her blood glucose in target. When the pancreas can't keep up with the extra demand for insulin, the blood glucose elevates, and gestational diabetes occurs. Generally this happens at about week 24 of the pregnancy, but it can happen sooner or possibly later in some women.

Unfortunately, when too much glucose builds up in the mother's blood, that glucose can affect the developing baby. Babies of moms who have gestational diabetes can become too big, which complicates delivery. These babies aren't born with diabetes, but they might be born with a low blood sugar level. They are also at risk for obesity and type 2 diabetes in later life.

The CDC estimates that gestational diabetes is present in 9.2 percent of pregnancies in the United States, and the rate of diabetes during pregnancy has been rising in recent years. Though the cause of gestational diabetes is not fully known, higher obesity rates may be contributing to this increase. Approximately 70 percent of women with gestational diabetes are overweight at the beginning of the pregnancy.

How Gestational Diabetes Is Diagnosed

Women are screened with a blood test during pregnancy for gestational diabetes. While guidelines for the screening, diagnosis, and treatment of gestational diabetes vary between organizations, the American Diabetes Association (ADA) recommends that a fasting (not eating for at least eight hours) blood glucose test be completed at the first prenatal visit to check for type 2 diabetes. If everything is okay, another test is not done until 24 to 28 weeks gestation. At that point in the pregnancy, a two-hour OGTT is recommended (see Chapter 1 for a refresher on OGTT). The diagnosis of gestational diabetes is made when any of the following blood glucose values are exceeded:

- Fasting: $\geq$92 mg/dL

- One hour: $\geq$180 mg/dL

- Two hours: $\geq$153 mg/dL

If one of the blood glucose results is above target, gestational diabetes is diagnosed. Good diabetes control is especially important during pregnancy to protect both the mother and the baby, so action should be taken right away when a diagnosis of gestational diabetes is made.

Does It Go Away After Pregnancy?

Most times the mom's blood glucose returns to normal after the baby is born. However, women who've had gestational diabetes have seven times the risk of developing type 2 diabetes in 5 to 10 years after the pregnancy. To rule out type 2 diabetes, an additional screening should be completed 6 to 12 weeks after delivery. Due to the increased risk for type 2 diabetes, it is recommended that women with a history of gestational diabetes continue to have screenings completed at least every three years throughout their lives.

DIABETES DECODED

If you had gestational diabetes during pregnancy, you have a greater risk of gestational diabetes in any additional pregnancies and an increased risk for type 2 diabetes. Continuing to follow the guidelines for meal planning you used during your pregnancy and getting (or staying) active right away makes it possible to prevent diabetes. So take action now!

Less-Common Types of Diabetes

While the most commonly recognized types of diabetes have already been reviewed, there are other types of diabetes that are less well known and may be mistaken for type 1 and/or type 2 diabetes. Therefore, it's a good idea to know about these different types, even though you may never meet anyone with these types of diabetes or hear about them again.

Latent Autoimmune Diabetes in Adults

Latent autoimmune diabetes in adults (LADA) more resembles type 1 diabetes and yet is often misdiagnosed and treated as type 2 diabetes because it generally occurs in people over age 30. Somewhere between type 1 and type 2 diabetes, it is also referred to as type 1 ½ diabetes. People with LADA have the autoantibodies seen in type 1 diabetes but often don't need insulin to control blood glucose until months or possibly years after diagnosis, similar to type 2. This is because rather than the rapid onset of type 1 diabetes, LADA progresses more slowly; however, eventually beta cells succumb to the autoimmune attack, and insulin is required for treatment. If a person is thin, doesn't show signs of insulin resistance, and doesn't have a family history of type 2 diabetes, LADA should be considered.

LADA may be significantly underrecognized, potentially making up 10 percent of all cases of type 2 diabetes. Why is it so commonly missed? There are no specific guidelines for antibody screening in "adult onset" diabetes, and if testing is never done, medical providers may not know autoantibodies are present. But as this type of diabetes becomes more recognized, testing might increase in patients fitting the description for LADA. Does it make a difference to know? It just might. Starting insulin therapy sooner rather than later may help to keep the beta cells working longer. If beta cells are preserved, it could potentially help limit diabetes complications down the road.

Another reason that a diagnosis of LADA matters is that new treatment options are constantly being developed to treat type 1 diabetes. If a new, successful option emerges, people with LADA may also benefit from the same strategies to treat type 1 diabetes.

Maturity-Onset Diabetes of the Young

What is maturity-onset diabetes of the young (MODY), you ask? Well, it's not type 1 diabetes and it's not type 2 diabetes, but it is often confused with one or the other. MODY is caused by a single *gene mutation* (monogenic), whereas type 1 and type 2 diabetes require multiple gene mutations (polygenic) and environmental triggers.

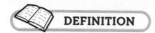 **DEFINITION**

> **Gene mutation** is a permanent alteration to the DNA sequence of a gene. Gene mutations can be inherited from one or both parents, or they can be acquired. Acquired mutations happen in the DNA of cells during a person's lifetime and are not passed on to the next generation. Changes can be triggered by environmental factors, such as ultraviolet radiation from the sun or DNA errors as it copies itself as cells divide.

MODY may be confused with type 1 diabetes when initially diagnosed because it generally presents in children, teens, and young adults. MODY may also be mislabeled as type 2 diabetes when it is not recognized until adulthood.

MODY should be suspected when considering a type 1 diabetes diagnosis but the following occurs:

- No autoantibodies are found, and the blood test results are negative.

- A person continues to produce a significant amount of insulin years beyond diagnosis.

MODY should be suspected when considering a type 2 diabetes diagnosis but the following occurs:

- A person is of normal weight or not significantly overweight and has no signs of insulin resistance.

- The person has a steady, mildly elevated blood glucose, and the symptoms are not consistent with type 1 or type 2 diabetes.

Another scenario where MODY should be explored is when the person is a member of a family where three or more successive generations have been diagnosed with diabetes. Genetic testing can aid in uncovering this type of diabetes. Diagnosing MODY correctly may make a difference in treatment options and could help to identify other family members as well.

Other Types and Causes of Diabetes

Diabetes may have a number of different causes, including other genetic diseases, damage to the pancreas, removal of the pancreas, endocrine diseases, autoimmune diseases, medications, chemicals, and toxins. These types of diabetes may either be unique to a health condition, or the health condition may trigger type 1 or type 2 diabetes. For instance, type 2 diabetes is more common in people with Down's syndrome, Turner syndrome, and Klinefelter syndrome than in the general population. The autoimmune disorder lupus erythematosus may also lead to type 1 diabetes. Trauma to the pancreas may result in surgical removal causing insulin dependent diabetes that is not the same as type 1 diabetes. So let's review some of the more common causes and types.

Pancreatitis

Pancreatitis is a condition where the pancreas becomes inflamed, which can lead to pancreatic damage. In addition to making insulin, the pancreas aids in digestion. When everything is working normally, the pancreas produces enzymes and moves them out to the small intestine, where they become active to help digest food. With pancreatitis, digestive enzymes become active while still inside the pancreas, causing pancreatic inflammation. Pancreatitis can be *acute* or *chronic*. Acute pancreatitis has a sudden onset and the inflammation only lasts for a short time. If acute pancreatitis occurs repeatedly, it can lead to chronic pancreatitis, and the likelihood of permanent harm to the pancreas goes up. Scar tissue can build up inside the pancreas, which can lead to irreversible damage of the insulin producing beta cells.

Acute pancreatitis can be caused by a number of things, including the following:

- Gallstones
- Alcoholism
- High triglycerides in the blood (blood fats)
- Cigarette smoking
- Cystic fibrosis
- Infection
- Injury

If someone has a family history of pancreatitis, they may be more susceptible to the condition.

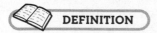 **DEFINITION**

> **Acute** refers to a condition with abrupt onset and rapid progression. Acute conditions are generally resolved with medical treatment. **Chronic** refers to a disease or condition that is persistent and long lasting. A chronic disease is generally not preventable by a vaccine or curable with medical treatment, so the goal of chronic disease is generally to manage it. Some chronic diseases like diabetes can be well managed and controlled.

Acute pancreatitis may range from uncomfortable to a severe, life-threatening emergency. Signs of acute pancreatitis may include upper abdominal pain, abdominal pain that wraps around to the back or gets worse after eating, fever, and nausea and/or vomiting. Being unable to get comfortable in any position or having severe abdominal pain and uncontrolled vomiting are signs that medical help is needed right away. Generally, people are able to recover completely from acute pancreatitis after receiving medical treatment; however, in severe cases, damage may not only be to the pancreas but other organs, such as the heart, lungs, and kidneys.

Symptoms of chronic pancreatitis are similar to acute pancreatitis. Some people may feel ongoing pain that may be disabling. Other symptoms include oily, smelly stools and losing weight without trying due to malabsorption of food caused by the lack of digestive enzymes. While other medical conditions can also cause these symptoms, it is best to seek advice from a medical provider if these symptoms occur and aren't going away.

Whether acute or chronic, the damage from pancreatitis can lead to insulin-dependent diabetes. The type of diabetes caused by damage from pancreatitis is not the same as type 1, where the damage to the pancreas is caused by autoantibodies, though both are treated with insulin. In addition to treating the diabetes, pancreatic enzymes need to be taken as a supplement to be able to properly digest and absorb food.

Cystic Fibrosis

Cystic fibrosis is a genetic disorder that may lead to cystic fibrosis–related diabetes (CFRD), a different type of diabetes than in people without cystic fibrosis. CFRD has characteristics of both type 1 and type 2 diabetes and is caused by unusually thick mucus that blocks the pancreas. This blockage leads to scarring inside the pancreas. CFRD becomes common in people with cystic fibrosis as they get older. According to the Cystic Fibrosis Foundation, 35 percent of people with cystic fibrosis ages 20 to 29 have CFRD, while a full 43 percent of people over age 30 have CFRD.

Insulin is required for treatment of CFRD. Due to the disorder itself, insulin resistance is also common among people with CFRD, as in type 2 diabetes. Screening for CFRD is recommended because many people with cystic fibrosis don't have any typical symptoms of diabetes. However, once insulin is started and blood glucose improves, people with CFRD start feeling better and other cystic fibrosis symptoms may also improve.

> **DID YOU KNOW?**
>
> Cystic fibrosis is a genetic disease that affects 30,000 people living in the United States. This life-threatening illness causes the body to produce thick, sticky mucus that clogs the lungs and obstructs the pancreas. Symptoms of cystic fibrosis include frequent lung infections, coughing, shortness of breath, difficulty gaining weight, and poor growth. This disease is usually diagnosed by age 2. About half of the population with cystic fibrosis is over age 18.

Chemicals and Medications

Exposure to some chemicals has been tentatively linked to the development of diabetes. For example, dioxin, a contaminant of Agent Orange, may be linked with type 2 diabetes. Due to this link, in 2000, a report issued by the Institute of Medicine (IOM) prompted the U.S. Department of Veterans Affairs (VA) to add type 2 diabetes to the list of "service connected" conditions. Veterans exposed to the herbicide Agent Orange during the Vietnam War may now be eligible for disability compensation and health care. The poison arsenic is also thought to be linked to diabetes.

Some medications are also thought to be connected to developing diabetes. Examples of medications that disrupt the action of insulin or impair beta cell function include drugs to treat human immunodeficiency virus (HIV) and certain psychiatric drugs. Corticosteroids—steroid drugs like prednisone, cortisone, and hydrocortisone—also make diabetes control more difficult because chemically they are similar to cortisol, also known as the "stress hormone." They are used to treat inflammation and suppress the immune system in conditions like arthritis, asthma and other breathing problems, severe allergies, and cancer. So just like the real thing, blood glucose and blood pressure can elevate—in addition to other side effects—in response to these medications. Blood glucose may be periodically monitored to catch elevated blood glucose early, and diabetes medications and/or insulin may be needed for treatment.

The Least You Need to Know

- Type 1 diabetes is an autoimmune disorder that cannot be prevented and requires taking insulin to sustain life. It comes on quickly and may cause a life-threatening condition called *diabetic ketoacidosis,* or DKA.

- LADA and MODY are two forms of diabetes that may be mistaken for type 1 and/or type 2 diabetes.

- Gestational diabetes is diagnosed during pregnancy. Mothers who have had gestational diabetes and their children are at higher risk of developing type 2 diabetes.

- Some types of diabetes may be caused by other autoimmune disorders, genetic diseases, damage to the pancreas, chemicals, or toxins.

Just the Facts: Dispelling Diabetes Misinformation

It seems everyone has something to say about diabetes. Information abounds on radio and television, in print, and on the internet. And when people find out you have diabetes, they often want to offer support. However, these sources may not always share the most accurate information. While much of what you hear may be potentially beneficial, you can easily come across material that is misleading at best and harmful at worst. How can you tell a false claim from sound advice?

In this chapter, we go over misinformation shared about diabetes and how you can get to the truth. By dispelling the myths and learning how to sort out fact from fiction, you can gain the knowledge to become a diabetes truth sleuth.

In This Chapter

- Debunking the most common diabetes myths
- What diabetes information can you trust on the internet?
- Links to helpful diabetes resources

Common Diabetes Myths

Myths involving diabetes include food and medical topics that may be offered up to people with diabetes as helpful when in fact they are just rumors filled with misleading information. These myths are dramatic to draw attention, and there is usually a ring of truth to them. They generally contain a warning or safety issue that makes people want to pass them on to others. In fact, some diabetes misinformation has been shared so frequently that many people believe it.

When you are faced with all the myths, the facts can become muddled and lost in the misconceptions. So let's debunk some of the myths and get you on the right path to managing your diabetes!

"You Should Eat Special Diabetic Foods"

It is a common belief that you have to give up all of your favorite foods and start eating diabetic or dietetic foods when you have diabetes. That is one huge myth! The fact is, so-called "diabetic foods" may not actually be healthier for you than the regular foods you choose. For instance, one small piece of chocolate or "fun-size" candy bar won't have much of an effect on your blood glucose. If you buy the diabetic or sugar-free version of the same type of candy, it may have more calories from fat and still have the same effect on your blood sugar as the regular versions.

 DIABETES DECODED

> Everyone has cravings for foods that are not the healthiest options. Because people with diabetes often think that all sweets need to be cut out of their diet, this often leads to wanting sugary treats even more. The best way to deal with cravings is to tell yourself it is okay to eat the foods you crave in small amounts. Once you know you can have any food when you really want it, it makes it easier to choose the healthier options most of the time.

The key when it comes to planning your meals and snacks when you have diabetes is moderation. One common problem with purchasing diabetic food is thinking you can eat more of it without any consequences. However, eating too many calories leads to weight gain, no matter where those calories are coming from. So if you eat more of the sugar-free food than you would have of the original food, you are likely taking in extra calories. Portions still count! Therefore, no matter what you decide to eat, you must keep in mind how much you're taking in at one sitting. Notice the example for chocolate was a small or fun-size serving. It is okay to include the foods you love in your eating plan—just not in unlimited amounts, and probably not every day. Enjoy a few bites of your favorite treat and savor the flavor. And by not purchasing all diabetic treats, you can save money, as specialty foods usually comes with a higher price tag.

"Eating Too Much Sugar Causes Diabetes"

This myth, which is generally associated with type 2 diabetes, doesn't necessarily have as simple an answer as you would like. You probably know that eating too much sugar is not healthy. Sugar doesn't provide any vitamins, minerals, fiber, or anything else that is beneficial to your health—just calories. Because lifestyle factors play a significant role in the development of type 2 diabetes, unhealthy food and beverage choices may lead to problems over time. For instance, sweetened beverages have been linked with increased health risks. Sugary drinks such as regular soda pop, sweet tea, sports drinks, and fruit punch have been associated not only with an increased risk of diabetes, but also heart disease. People who drink at least one to two cans of soda each day are 26 percent more likely to develop type 2 diabetes and have a 20 percent increased risk of having a heart attack than those who rarely include these beverages.

However, simply drinking sugary drinks or eating sugary foods won't cause diabetes. Without a genetic predisposition to diabetes, empty calorie choices alone do not trigger diabetes. Still, you give yourself the best chance of avoiding or managing diabetes by making healthy choices. If those sweetened drinks I mentioned are part of your daily routine, now is a good time to make a change. What should you drink instead? A nice, tall glass of water would be a great choice!

 DIABETES DECODED

Water, anyone? Replacing even one soda with a glass of water can save you hundreds of calories and many teaspoons of sugar. One 12-ounce can of regular soda has 150 calories and 10 teaspoons of sugar, while one 20-ounce bottle of soda packs a high-calorie punch at 239 calories and a whopping 17 teaspoons of sugar!

"Being Overweight Causes Diabetes"

While being overweight is a major risk factor for type 2 diabetes, the truth is that many people who are overweight never develop type 2 diabetes. Some people with type 2 diabetes are a normal weight or only slightly overweight. A combination of genetic and lifestyle factors are what lead to the development of type 2 diabetes. Family history, age, and ethnicity also play a part. Still, while being overweight does not stand alone as a cause for diabetes, it is a good idea to know your weight status.

The CDC uses the body mass index (BMI) to measure weight in the population. The BMI weight status categories are the same for all adults 20 years and older and for both men and women. The following table shows BMI compared to weight status.

Weight Status Based on BMI

BMI	Weight Status
Below 18.5	Underweight
18.5 to 24.9	Normal
25 to 29.9	Overweight
30 and above	Obese

Source: CDC

People with "normal" weight status tend to be the healthiest. "Overweight" and "obese" are labels for weight that is above what is considered healthy for a given height. In adults, overweight and obesity weight ranges are determined by using height and weight to calculate BMI. For most people, BMI tracks along with body fat—the higher the body fat, the higher the BMI. The BMI is also an indicator of health risk. The greater the number, the more likely certain diseases and health problems will occur.

So how do you figure out your BMI? All you need is your height and weight. The official formula is as follows:

$$BMI = weight\ (kg) \div height^2\ (m)$$

Not a big fan of the metric system? Here's another way to calculate your BMI using your weight in pounds and your height in inches:

$$BMI = [weight \div height^2] \times 703$$

To give you an idea of how this formula works, the following is how you find the BMI of a 150-pound person who is 5 feet 7 inches tall (67 inches):

$$150 \div 67^2 = .033$$

$$.033 \times 703 = 24$$

If you are not a fan of math and want to skip the calculations altogether, there are many websites that offer BMI calculators and charts, including the CDC (cdc.gov/healthyweight/assessing/bmi/adult_BMI/english_bmi_calculator/bmi_calculator.html). On these sites, you can simply type in your height and weight and let the calculator do the number crunching for you. Your medical provider can also tell you what your BMI is if you're not sure.

If you find you're overweight and have known risk factors for diabetes, losing weight should be a top priority. Even if you don't have type 2 risk factors, however, positive changes in your eating and physical activity now may have a big payoff by preventing other health problems down the road.

"If You Don't Eat Right, You Will Have to Start Insulin"

This is another whopper! If you have type 2 diabetes, you don't always have to take insulin to manage it; therefore, starting insulin may seem like a bad thing. Sometimes this myth sounds like a threat—"You'd better eat right or else"—where the punishment ("or else") is taking insulin. However, you are not a failure if you have to take insulin to control your blood sugar.

 FOR YOUR SAFETY

> When you have diabetes, it is nearly impossible to keep your blood glucose in the target range 100 percent of the time. However, if your blood glucose is *staying* out of range, talk with your medical provider right away. You may need to change how you manage your diabetes.

Insulin is really just another tool to help control your blood glucose when you need it. Sometimes insulin is used briefly to control type 2 diabetes after the initial diagnosis, when you are sick, or possibly when you are in the hospital. After those situations resolve, you may be able to return to managing your diabetes with other medications. Or if you have had type 2 diabetes for a long time, the beta cells in your pancreas may no longer be able to make enough insulin, making it imperative to take insulin. If taking insulin gets your blood glucose into a healthy range, it is definitely a good thing. So don't put off taking insulin when you need it just because you think you'll eat better in the future.

"Healthy Foods Don't Raise Blood Sugar"

Many healthy foods contain *carbohydrates,* which are processed by your body into sugar. Foods with carbohydrates include any that have starch or sugar in them. For instance, foods such as whole grains, low-fat and nonfat milk and yogurt, fruit, dried beans and lentils, and starchy vegetables like sweet potatoes contain quality carbohydrates. These nutrient-rich foods are recommended for a healthy diabetes eating plan. However, if eaten in large amounts, these same foods may certainly raise your blood sugar. Because your body doesn't know the difference between naturally occurring sugar from grapes or added sugars in the form of candy like jelly beans, for example, both can raise your blood sugar too high. On the flip side, if the amount of carbohydrates you eat is matched to the insulin you are making (or taking), neither food will raise your blood sugar too high.

The goal of a diabetes meal plan is not to avoid carbohydrates, but to balance them with available insulin to keep blood glucose in a healthy range most of the time. While both healthy and unhealthy foods can raise your blood sugar, it's best to choose foods that contain vitamins, minerals, and fiber, which are more beneficial to your health than foods filled with added sugars.

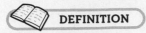 **DEFINITION**

Carbohydrates (or carbs) are one of the main components in food. Carbohydrates are broken down into glucose, which the body uses for energy.

As Seen on the Internet

If it's on the internet, it must be true, right? That question is easily answered with a resounding no! A quick search on the internet using the keyword "diabetes" yields millions of results in a fraction of a second. How can you possibly sort diabetes fact from fiction with the ridiculously huge amount of information available? The following are a few key tips that will help you sort out the good, the bad, and the downright ugly on the net.

Internet Content Warning Signs

Have you ever heard the saying "If it sounds too good to be true, it probably is"? This is applicable to many things, but when applied to diabetes, certain claims should tip you off right away. The following are some common signs the diabetes content you've found on the internet is untrustworthy:

- If it claims a product can "cure diabetes" without you having to do anything except take the product, it is definitely not valid.

- When a product claims to control a whole laundry list of symptoms, consider it a red flag. For example, if the promoters claim it treats everything from athlete's foot to zinc deficiency and everything in between, you know it doesn't really work. If it did, everyone would be using it!

- An assertion that there are absolutely no risks or side effects is also highly questionable. Alert bells should definitely be ringing!

- Diet programs that promise you will lose weight within a certain period of time—for example, "lose 10 pounds in 10 days"—are not credible sources. There are no guarantees for weight loss, and not everyone loses weight in the same amount of time. Some people may not lose weight at all. Legitimate programs won't make those type of promises.

- If a website is filled with multiple testimonials and personal stories but no facts or data, there probably are no real facts to report.

- Beware of websites promising free information about diabetes that tell you next to nothing, and then prompt you to enroll or sign up to get the full scoop. If you're asked to start entering a lot of personal information about yourself, steer clear.

- Prompts that say you must "act now" to get the deal they're offering are designed to trigger you to make an impulse purchase. Don't let marketers make a decision for you. Take some time to think about it. You can check other websites to see whether it really is a good deal.

But it may not actually be the content of the article or paper that's misleading. Many times, a headline may be the culprit by only telling part of the story. For instance, a headline stating "Medical Breakthrough: A Cure for Diabetes" sounds amazing. This would make most people want to be the first in line for whatever this cure might be. However, the rest of the article may go on to describe that this discovery is a cure solely for type 1 diabetes, and the study was done with mice, not humans. While any potential cure for diabetes, even in mice, is very promising research that should be shared with the public, that doesn't mean people can go to the corner pharmacy to fill a prescription or undergo a simple, low-risk procedure to be cured anytime soon. So rather than jumping to conclusions after reading a headline or hearing a sound bite, it is a good idea to explore a bit further to verify the information.

FOR YOUR SAFETY

Never stop taking your insulin or other diabetes medication in favor of a product you heard about through the internet or another source. Any changes in your medication, including adding an over-the-counter remedy, should be discussed with your medical provider first. Some herbal remedies, supplements, and natural medicines can interact with your prescription medications, making them either more or less effective. Even though increased effectiveness sounds positive, sometimes it can lead to toxic levels of a medication in your body.

Sources of Reputable Information About Diabetes

One way to verify if there is merit to any claims about diabetes is to check a trustworthy website to see if there is additional discussion on the topic. Fortunately, there are many reliable sources of information about diabetes; you just have to know what to look for. The web address itself can give you a good idea that you are on the right track; look for .org, .gov, and .edu to identify trusted information on the web.

Websites ending in .org are used by many nonprofit organizations (though others can register a website as .org, so be a bit cautious). The following are some .org sites you can explore for accurate information on diabetes:

- American Diabetes Association (diabetes.org)
- Academy of Nutrition and Dietetics (eatright.org)
- Juvenile Diabetes Research Foundation (jdrf.org)

Government websites are the ones you'll find ending in .gov. The following .gov websites have a wealth of information related to diabetes and healthful eating:

- National Diabetes Education Program (ndep.nih.gov)

- Choose My Plate (choosemyplate.gov)

- Centers for Disease Control and Prevention (cdc.gov/diabetes)

Websites ending in .edu indicate academic institutions. These .edu sites are great resources for health-related issues, including diabetes:

- Harvard School of Public Health (hsph.harvard.edu/nutritionsource/)

- University of Georgia Cooperative Extension Service (extension.uga.edu)

- University of Illinois Extension (urbanext.illinois.edu/diabetes2/intro.cfm)

 DIABETES DECODED

> The key to sorting out whether you can trust a .com website is the source of the content. Mainstream research studies and well-known scientific literature will be included as sources. Not only will the top sites have contributors that are medical doctors and other qualified health-care providers like registered nurses, registered dietitian nutritionists, and certified diabetes educators, they also list the experts' backgrounds and training. It is one thing to have information provided by an MD, but if that MD has a great deal of experience in diabetes and is employed by a well-respected institution, the information is much more likely to be credible. The best websites will also have a group of expert reviewers and advisors to provide increased accuracy. WebMD (webmd.com) and dLife (dlife.com) are two such .com websites.

Beyond these links, you can also check out Appendix B of this book, which contains links to many useful websites to help you successfully manage your diabetes.

For those instances when you're simply exploring the internet or checking your email and come across diabetes information, there are a number of websites dedicated to fact checking. The Snopes website (snopes.com) is well known for sleuthing out the facts in the forwarded emails lurking in your inbox. You can either type the topic in their search bar or check out the "Food" and "Medical" categories for information on diabetes. Another website, Quackwatch (quackwatch. com), is specifically dedicated to identifying medical quackery and health fraud. One of the sections on the website even discusses the different ploys used by fraudulent promoters of cure-alls and "natural" products. Check out the "Tips for Navigating Our Web Sites" link on their front page, and then get searching!

The Least You Need to Know

- Misinformation and myths about diabetes may be passed on by others because they believe the information is true or they simply want you to buy their product.
- You can find helpful information on the internet if you check for reputable sources and read past the headlines.
- Check the facts using reliable websites before you pass on an email that sounds like it is a bit too far-fetched to be true.
- A list of resources is available in Appendix B of this book to help you with your quest for truthful information about diabetes management.

Putting Yourself on the Right Path

To be successful in self-managing your diabetes, you have to make positive behavior changes. That may seem easier said than done, but in this part, we help you get into the right mind-set to make those changes. We discuss the importance of understanding the motivations behind your decisions, the SMART method of setting goals, and the ways you can measure your progress.

When you have diabetes, you also need to have support—personally and medically—for your efforts. Therefore, in this part, we identify the critical health-care professionals to include on your team, as well as how your family and friends can help. While we know it's tough to depend on others, especially when you don't automatically get the kind of help you need, we show you how you can communicate to gain the type of support you want to receive.

We close this part with ways you can prevent and treat both short-term and long-term problems caused by diabetes. You discover when and how to handle situations on your own, and when you need to seek medical help from others.

How to Make Changes for Diabetes Management

In the first part of the book, you learned why it is important to manage diabetes well and keep your blood glucose in a target range. However, you are probably already aware from past experience that *knowing* what's necessary doesn't necessarily equal *doing* what's necessary—making that leap from knowledge to action is the hard part.

Because diabetes self-management requires certain behaviors along with frequent decision making, this chapter focuses on helping you make behavior changes to achieve the best possible diabetes control. By using the right resources and understanding what motivates you to make positive behavior changes, that leap from knowledge to action will become easier for you.

In This Chapter

- Identifying why you want to make changes
- Understanding the importance of goal setting
- Tools to help make positive behavior changes
- Sustaining change

Making Changes Based on the AADE7

The American Association of Diabetes Educators (AADE) has identified seven categories of self-care behaviors called the *AADE7* that you can use as a framework to effectively manage your diabetes. The AADE7 categories are: healthy eating, being active, monitoring, taking medication, problem solving, reducing risks, and healthy coping. Increasing skills in these areas of self-care have been demonstrated to predict good outcomes for people with diabetes. The following walks you through what each of the seven categories means for you:

Healthy eating: By choosing the right amount of food at the right times, you can achieve or maintain a healthy weight and manage your blood glucose. Making healthful food choices most of the time also helps decrease health risks associated with diabetes.

Being active: You should include physical activity in your regular routine. Aerobic activities (such as bicycling, jogging, walking, or swimming), as well as stretching and strength training are all ways to be active that are beneficial to your health. Being physically active can help keep your heart healthy, help you manage your weight, and improve your blood glucose control.

 DIABETES DECODED

Remember, when changing a behavior, start with where you are now. For example, if you are currently inactive, starting with a walk to your mailbox and back four days a week may be an appropriate initial goal for you. You can then gradually build on your success and add in more activity as you progress.

Monitoring: Testing your blood glucose regularly lets you know if things are working well, or if changes are needed. Sharing your blood glucose results with your medical provider allows for additional assessment to determine if your diabetes medications are working effectively.

Taking medication: While you may or may not need diabetes medications initially, the longer you have type 2 diabetes, the more likely it is that you will need diabetes medications and/or insulin. Taking your medication and/or insulin appropriately and knowing how to balance it with food and physical activity is an important skill.

Problem solving: Because diabetes is chronic, and many everyday activities affect blood glucose, problem-solving skills are used on a regular basis. Knowing how to respond if your blood glucose is too high or too low, or if your routine is going to be different than usual, is essential for optimal diabetes control.

Reducing risks: Knowing and understanding what tests and exams need to be done and making regular visits to your medical provider are things you can do to reduce your risk of diabetes complications. Examples of preventive care include eye exams, blood pressure checks, lab tests (A1C, cholesterol, triglycerides, and urine protein), and foot exams.

Healthy coping: Diabetes self-management is challenging and complex. Feelings like being hassled, overwhelmed, angry, out of control, sad, and stressed are common. Diabetes not only affects you physically, but emotionally as well. Being able to cope with these feelings and maintain ongoing motivation is critical in not letting diabetes take over your life but instead empowering you to overcome it!

Getting on the Path to Change

Did reading through the previous categories seem a bit overwhelming and make you feel like you have to change everything you're currently doing? That's not the case. You're probably doing a number of things well already, so you certainly don't have to change everything. Also, relearning and changing your behaviors is a process; you'll be making gradual changes over time, not jumping into major changes straight off. So how can you get on the path to managing your diabetes?

Assessing Your Motivation

Relearning and changing your behavior is absolutely possible, but it's certainly not easy! Not many people want to make a change just for the sake of change itself. If you don't know what you're going to get out of it, it probably won't happen. It also helps if you are making a change that is your choice—something that you *want* to do rather than something that you *should* or *have* to do. Therefore, it is a good idea to assess your *motivation* before getting started. Taking a step back and asking yourself a few questions before you dive into making changes will help you focus on where to start and decide exactly what you want to accomplish.

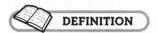 **DEFINITION**

Motivation is an internal process that initiates, directs, and maintains behaviors. It can cause you to take action and to move toward a certain goal.

A sense of importance and confidence about making a change helps drive motivation. The following can help you determine whether you're ready to make a change:

Ask yourself whether the change is important to you. If the change feels like something you really want to do and there's a sense of urgency about making the change, it's a good place to start. However, if you just don't feel it is important, you may want to move on to something else for now. It might just not be the right time to make that particular change.

Ask yourself how confident you are about making the change. Note that we're not asking you to determine whether the change is easy; you simply need to decide whether it's something you feel you're able to do. Belief in your ability to make a change helps motivate you to get started. If you feel it is impossible, even if you're motivated, it will be very difficult to make that particular change. For instance, even if you feel it is important to increase your exercise but you just hate to exercise and really can't picture yourself exercising, start with something else so you don't just give up.

The great thing about choosing something that you think is important and feel you can accomplish, and then accomplishing it, is that it builds confidence. And once you have that confidence, you'll want to make more changes for your well-being. That's how motivation can help you manage your health and stay on track when you have diabetes.

Making Long-Term and Sustainable Changes

To make long-lasting changes in behavior for your health, there needs to be a long-term, sustainable benefit. It may seem like avoiding something negative, such as diabetes complications, should be enough. But fear only works initially; it doesn't keep you on track in the long run. For instance, if you experienced a heart attack, you may decide to give up all fried foods and never use salt again. But once that fear of being rushed to the emergency room has subsided, the extreme changes in eating habits may not seem so urgent. And because you applied an all-or-nothing approach, it is not very sustainable—even if you eat fried food one time, the goal has failed. If, on the other hand, your long-term goal is to be healthier and more active so you can play with your grandchildren, now you're getting somewhere. That is something you can work toward and build upon in the future, and you're not setting yourself up for failure by defining success in a narrow window (unlike the never eating fried foods example). Plus, by connecting it to something important in your life—your grandchildren—you're adding something personally meaningful to the change.

Another way to incentivize yourself to practice new behaviors over the long term is to plan rewards. In order for these to work effectively, rewards should be something you like that reinforce the new behavior. For instance, if you've taken up walking to improve your health, put some money in a jar each time you walk to save up for nicer walking shoes. If you want the new shoes, you're more likely to stick with it.

However, don't fall into the trap of using food for a reward. For example, after you saw the word *reward*, you may have thought about rewarding yourself with a hot fudge sundae or some other treat. The problem with that is that it doesn't reinforce a positive behavior when it comes to your health. While you can enjoy a treat on occasion, you should not use it as a reward. It's all about promoting a sustainable, healthy lifestyle.

FOR YOUR SAFETY

Making a sudden, extreme change in your eating habits or physical activity level is not recommended and may lead to hypoglycemia. This is especially true if you are taking certain diabetes medications and/or insulin. For instance, cutting out all carbohydrate and exercising four hours a day after being sedentary may lower your blood glucose, but not in a safe way. This type of change is not good for diabetes management or for your overall health. When in doubt, talk it over with your medical provider.

Setting Goals

Common reasons that people can't make sustainable changes are that they are vague about what they want to accomplish and they don't have a plan. If you set out to make a change such as "eat less" or "test blood sugar more," how would you know if these changes are achieved effectively? It is difficult to measure progress or say a change is successful unless you set a goal. So now that you've identified a behavior you'd like to change that is important, possible, and has a meaningful benefit, let's look at what you need to do to set a goal!

Being SMART About Goal Setting

To help you develop a goal that will work for you, use the SMART goal-setting principles (a sample SMART goal-setting worksheet is included in Appendix C). A SMART goal is broken down as the following:

- **Specific:** A specific goal has a better chance of success.

- **Measurable:** Measuring your progress can help you stay on track.

- **Action-oriented:** A goal should be able to be broken down into smaller action steps.

- **Realistic:** It should be a goal you feel you can start working on now.

- **Timely:** Have a time frame that specifies a beginning and an end.

Let's walk through how to turn a common diabetes management goal into a SMART goal. Here's an example of a goal many people with diabetes want to achieve:

Goal: "I want to lose weight."

This particular goal isn't specific or measurable, there are no steps listed on how to work toward the goal, and there is no indication about when this will happen.

The first step is to figure out the expected benefit. Why do you want to lose weight?

> "I want to lose weight to be able to easily walk up several flights of stairs without being short of breath."

Here is the revised goal using SMART goal-setting principles:

> "I will lose five pounds over the next six weeks by taking my lunch to work three days a week and choosing vegetables for my evening snack."

As you can see, the goal is specific (losing 5 pounds), measurable (weighing yourself gives you feedback on your progress), action-oriented (taking a lunch three days a week and eating vegetables every evening), realistic (the goal is challenging but still achievable), and timely (happening over a six-week time frame).

 DIABETES DECODED

While it is important for a goal to be realistic, it shouldn't be so easy that you could do it without really trying. Give yourself a goal that is a bit of a stretch—one that challenges you.

Giving It a Chance

In order to learn new behaviors, you have to "unlearn" the habits and beliefs that are keeping you away from what you want to achieve. Your current habits and beliefs have been learned and practiced. You develop your own unique filter with which you see things based on your life experience. That's why new behaviors must also be practiced for some time until they become habits.

When starting out with something new, it is best to try it for two weeks before deciding it's not for you. That way, you can make a more educated decision about how you would modify it or what you might do in place of it. Behavior change is a process; it's not a "one time and you're done" type of thing. Remember, it took a long time to learn your current behavior, so allow yourself time to learn the new healthful behavior.

Choosing smaller action steps and not just focusing on the end result can help you be more patient with yourself and your progress. While it is easy to get frustrated, don't be harder on yourself than you would with someone else. Think about what you would tell a friend trying to make similar changes, and then tell yourself the same thing.

However, if you find after some time and patience that the goal still seems unreasonable, feel free to make some alterations or even find something new to replace it. Let's look at an example of when modifying a goal might be needed.

Current goal: Walk for 30 minutes in the neighborhood after work on Monday, Wednesday, and Friday.

If you've committed to walk but the weather has been so bad that you haven't been able to venture outside, modification is in order. In this example, the only thing that needs to be changed is the location. You could start walking at an indoor location such as your local mall.

Revised goal: Walk for 30 minutes at the mall after work on Monday, Wednesday, and Friday.

As you can see, goals aren't set in stone; you can modify what you're doing and still continue on the path of managing your diabetes. Practice may not make perfect, but it can help you establish new, healthy habits!

Tools and Strategies to Keep You On Track

There are many tools available to help you with your diabetes self-management goals. Let's take a look at how you can best keep records of your progress, evaluate what has worked for you, make changes that align with your lifestyle, and bust through any barriers you have.

 DIABETES DECODED

The area of focus for your change may determine the best place to look for help. For instance, if you want to quit smoking, an excellent resource is the smokefree.gov website. Need to reduce your stress? Harvard Medical School has free stress reduction resources available on their website health.harvard.edu/topic/stress. Public libraries are also a great place to find free resources. You can even use the resources provided in Appendix B. Whatever you decide, you'll be amazed at what is available once you start looking!

Keeping Records

A way to know how a change is affecting you—and to keep yourself honest—is to maintain records of what you're doing. For example, people who keep food and blood glucose records tend to have better diabetes control because it provides a full picture of how certain foods can affect their blood glucose. Just testing your blood glucose and putting the meter away doesn't help if you never do anything with the information. Writing down your blood glucose results, along with foods eaten, allows you to see a pattern to your results and identify where changes are needed. (We talk more about how to keep blood glucose records in Chapter 11.)

Keeping track of your physical activity also helps with meeting your exercise goals. When you measure the time (number of minutes) and frequency (number of days per week) of your exercise, it reinforces a sense of accomplishment. And if you're not quite meeting your exercise goal, your records will help you figure out why. Records like these can provide an objective measure for your progress.

If you just can't bring yourself to write your records on paper, there are many tracking tools that are available for use with computers, cell phones, and other mobile devices that can make record keeping easier. The following are a few we'd recommend (see Appendixes B and C for more ways to keep records):

- **MyFitnessPal (myfitnesspal.com):** You can track your food and activity with this. Their large food database makes it easy to enter the foods you've eaten.

- **MyFoodAdvisor (tracker.diabetes.org):** Plan meals, find recipes, set goals, and track your food and activity.

- **Supertracker (supertracker.usda.gov):** Track your food, activity, and weight management.

Whatever you decide to use, the information you gather should be able to help guide your diabetes management decisions. You can even take your records to your medical appointments for review; that way, your doctor can make informed decisions about potential changes in medication.

Evaluating What Has Worked for You

In the past, you've probably made some successful changes and some that were not so successful. Take a minute to think about those changes you made using the following questions:

- What actions led to positive change?

- What motivated you?

- How did you address your barriers?

- Could you identify the benefits to making the change?

- Did you understand the risks of not changing?

- Why do you think you achieved or didn't achieve what you set out to do?

Learning lessons from the past is a useful strategy for future change. Sometimes all you need to do is to make up your mind and decide to change!

DIABETES DECODED

Your attitude really makes a difference in your ability to successfully make a change. A negative attitude will almost always assure failure, while a positive attitude will take you a long way on the path to success. Be more aware of your thoughts and replace negative thoughts with positive statements, as if you've already achieved your goal. Statements such as "I am a successful diabetes manager" or "I am in control of my diabetes" are examples of positive statements.

Making Changes Compatible with Your Lifestyle

Because diabetes is an ongoing, chronic condition, it is important to make diabetes management work with your lifestyle. You are a person who happens to have diabetes; diabetes does not define you. Therefore, if you frame changes with your lifestyle in mind, you'll be making healthier decisions that don't compromise what makes you feel most comfortable.

For instance, maybe the word *exercise* brings up images of pain and misery, making it something that's obviously not high on your list. However, you have heard exercise is something that you "should do" because you have diabetes, so you are thinking about it. Looking at it in a way that fits into your lifestyle might just make it more achievable. How about something fun? If you like dancing, taking dance lessons with a friend might be something you would enjoy. Suddenly *exercise* becomes a fun activity—something you might choose to do. The payoff in this example is increasing physical activity while having fun with a friend and learning new dance moves. By making these types of choices, you can manage your diabetes and live a healthier life with success and satisfaction!

Busting Barriers

Everyone experiences barriers to change. And everyone who tries to make a change will experience a setback at some point. But that doesn't mean you should give up and throw in the towel. Defining the problem is the first step to get moving forward again. If you can figure out why you ran into a particular barrier, you can start to fix the problem. Here are a few questions that may help you identify and move past a barrier:

- What are your feelings about this problem?

- How will you feel if things don't change?

- What are your thoughts about this problem?

- What might help you think differently about this problem?

As you can see from the previous questions, it's about moving from a more subjective to a more objective mind-set with the issues—from feelings to thoughts. While it is true that you may not be able to fully change your feelings about the problem, if you reframe your thoughts and think about the problem in a new way, it can help you overcome it. For example, it would be very easy to feel that it is not fair that you have to test your blood glucose multiple times a day and just stop testing. But if you reframe it with the thinking that blood glucose monitoring provides you valuable feedback to manage your diabetes and stay healthy, you can get back on track.

However, there are times when your initial plan just has to be modified. In those cases, a backup plan that acknowledges barriers helps with long-term success. As an example, if your physical activity plan has been walking around your neighborhood in the evening, that may have worked wonderfully in the spring and summer. But when bad weather sets in, you may have to modify that plan by choosing a different activity. On those bad-weather days, a Plan B could be something like riding a stationary bike indoors, using an exercise video, or walking up and down the stairs in your house. By having an alternative, you allow yourself some flexibility so the barrier doesn't completely block you from staying on the path to good diabetes management.

The Least You Need to Know

- There are certain self-care behaviors—healthy eating, being active, monitoring, taking medication, problem solving, reducing risks, and healthy coping—that help you successfully manage your diabetes.
- Before you can change a behavior, you have to address what motivates the change and how sustainable it is.
- Setting SMART (specific, measurable, action-oriented, realistic, and timely) goals can help you make behavior changes that are possible but still challenging.
- Practicing your newly learned behavior is essential to making it a habit.
- Choose changes that work with your lifestyle.

Finding Care and Support

Once you've made up your mind to start managing your diabetes, you want to do it right and get the best possible results. Having medical care and personal support are wonderful ways to help you achieve your goals.

Because it can be confusing to figure out who does what in the medical field, this chapter reviews the roles of diabetes care team members, unravels how to identify knowledgeable experts, and discusses what type of help you can expect from the experts once you find them. We also talk about how people in your personal life can support your diabetes management, as well as what to do when you aren't getting the proper support from others. With a winning support system lined up on your side, you will be well on your way to becoming a diabetes manager extraordinaire!

In This Chapter

- Members of your diabetes care team
- What your diabetes care team can do for you
- Asking for help from family, friends, and co-workers

Creating a Diabetes Care Team

Because there are so many components to managing diabetes, sometimes it is difficult to remember them all, let alone excel at them. That is where your team comes in. There are various roles that each team member fills to support you in your efforts, whether it's additional assistance with medical management, nutrition, diabetes self-care skills, behavior change, and more. The team will work with you to develop an individualized plan that is unique to you.

Leading the Team

Before we get into the different experts that make up your team, though, let's start with the core of the team: you. As the person with diabetes, you are the leader—the captain of the team, the star of the show, the one in the driver's seat. Unfortunately, you can't give away the responsibility to manage your diabetes any more than you can give your diabetes away. However, you have the power to be the deciding factor on what's best for you. After all, you are the expert on you; you'll be the first to notice anything when it comes to your body. You decide what you're able, willing, and choose to actually do. Deciding what you'll eat, if you'll take your medication and/or insulin as prescribed, and if you're going to be physically active is also up to you. You have the responsibility of checking your blood glucose to see if it is all working or identifying where changes are needed. (Wow, that's a lot; no wonder you need a team!)

As the captain, you are actively involved in daily decision making and changing and modifying your plan. While the team can't be there with you the moment you are choosing whether or not you will eat a cookie or take the stairs instead of the elevator, with appropriate education from your team of experts, you can make informed decisions and have a better understanding of how your actions will affect your diabetes control.

 DIABETES DECODED

You are your own best advocate when it comes to your medical care. To get the most out of your visit to your team of experts, write out your top two or three questions and bring them with you to the appointment. It's best to focus on the ones that are most important to you; that way, you won't forget to ask them and you'll have time for the critical questions. If you go in with a laundry list of questions, it is difficult to stay on track and you might run out of time. When your provider asks you questions in return, be honest and do not hold back pertinent information. Not answering truthfully or only reporting the part you think the provider wants to hear only hurts you. The right medical decisions can't be made if the information you share isn't accurate.

Primary Care Provider

Generally, primary care providers are physicians with an internal medicine or family practice background. Mid-level medical providers, such as nurse practitioners and physician assistants who work in conjunction with physicians, are also increasingly becoming primary care providers. Your primary care provider generally oversees all of your medical care and makes referrals to other team members and specialists as needed.

If you're currently looking for a provider who accepts your insurance, it is best to find one who sees a number of patients with diabetes and is comfortable with the medical management of diabetes. It is important that you feel you can talk with your provider about health concerns and that you can ask questions to clarify anything you don't understand.

The following are some questions we suggest you ask your primary care provider or potential primary care provider about diabetes, as well as the answers you should be looking for:

- **What percentage of the patients you see have diabetes?** If the potential provider only sees a handful of patients with diabetes, it may be best to find someone with more experience in diabetes management.

- **What tests do you order for your patients with diabetes? How often are they ordered?** You can use the Diabetes Care Measures chart in Appendix C to see which tests are recommended by the ADA and how often they should be completed. If the potential provider states he uses the ADA standards, that means he follows ADA recommendations for appropriate medical tests.

- **Do you work with other diabetes professionals here in your office? If not, do you refer to endocrinologists, diabetes educators, and dietitians?** Look for a medical provider who refers to diabetes educators, registered dietitians, and endocrinologists when needed. It's not necessary to have diabetes educators and registered dietitians on site in the same office, but that makes it convenient for you.

- **What targets do you recommend for my diabetes management?** Ask about what your blood glucose, blood pressure, and cholesterol targets should be and what references the potential provider uses to determine those targets. If the provider isn't familiar with treatment targets, it's best to talk with someone else.

By being on the same page with your primary care provider, you ensure the information the rest of your team will receive from your provider will be in line with what you want and need.

Endocrinologist

Not everyone with diabetes—in particular, people with well-controlled type 2 diabetes—sees an *endocrinologist*. However, if your diabetes is not as well-controlled as you'd like and the standard management isn't working, it could be the time to request a referral to one. An endocrinologist is a doctor who specializes in diagnosis and treatment of conditions involving the *endocrine system*. Endocrinologists are board-certified internal medicine physicians who have met extra training and practice requirements in endocrinology and have passed a national standardized exam. Physicians who have accomplished this are board-certified in endocrinology, diabetes, and metabolism. While some endocrinologists specialize in diabetes, some choose to specialize in another specific area of the endocrine system (such as the reproductive system). In addition to treating diabetes, most endocrinologists treat conditions like hypothyroidism, Cushing's syndrome, osteoporosis, and Addison's disease.

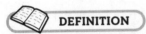 **DEFINITION**

> An **endocrinologist** is a physician who specializes in disorders of the endocrine system. Some endocrinologists are diabetes specialists. The **endocrine system** is a collection of glands that regulates metabolism, reproduction, growth, mood, sleep, and other body functions.

Endocrinologists who specialize in diabetes are familiar with the nuances of diabetes management and how to individualize treatment targets. They keep up to date on new diabetes treatment options and can work with you to develop more effective management strategies. Also, if you are dealing with diabetes complications, the additional training and experience of endocrinologists are helpful in giving you the information needed to make your decisions on the best course of action to improve your quality of life.

Diabetes Educator

Diabetes educators are health-care professionals specially trained to help people with diabetes learn self-care skills, achieve behavior change goals, and improve their health status. The majority of diabetes educators are registered nurses (RNs) and registered dietitians (RDs). However, diabetes educators may also be pharmacists, physical therapists, psychologists, podiatrists, and other qualified health-care professionals. Diabetes educators can be found in hospitals, physician offices, clinics, pharmacies, and community settings. Look for diabetes educators in recognized or accredited diabetes education programs.

You may have seen the CDE credential listed after a health-care professional's name. The letters CDE stand for Certified Diabetes Educator; this is an additional certification that diabetes educators can obtain. To become a CDE, a diabetes educator has to hold an eligible professional designation, such as RN or RD, have 1,000 hours of experience providing diabetes self-management education, meet additional training requirements, and pass a national exam. If you see "CDE," you can be confident that the health-care professional has knowledge and experience in working with people with diabetes.

A diabetes educator can help you learn how to do the following:

- Test your blood glucose and know what to do with the results
- Understand how your diabetes medications work
- Inject insulin
- Fit physical activity into your lifestyle
- Treat hypoglycemia
- Make healthier food choices

As you can see from this list, diabetes educators focus on helping you with real-life situations and the day-to-day aspects of diabetes care. This education is usually offered by them in classes or as individual sessions, with problem-solving skills and making healthier choices key areas discussed. Diabetes educators also coordinate your care with your provider so you benefit from a comprehensive diabetes management plan. Most insurance plans and Medicare cover diabetes education; you need a referral from your medical provider for diabetes self-management education to be covered by insurance.

DID YOU KNOW?

Diabetes educators and other health-care professionals can also be board-certified in advanced diabetes management (BC-ADM). To be eligible, health-care professionals must hold a Master's degree or higher and be an RN, RD, pharmacist, physician assistant, or physician. Also required for this certification are a minimum of 500 advanced clinical practice hours face-to-face with diabetes patients and passing a national exam.

Registered Dietitian Nutritionist

The Academy of Nutrition and Dietetics states "all registered dietitians are nutritionists, but not all nutritionists are registered dietitians." Therefore, the Academy recently approved an option for professionals who hold the RD credential to include the word *nutritionist* after registered dietitian, abbreviated as RDN. The rigorous requirements to become credentialed as an RDN are exactly the same as for the RD. RDs have a minimum of a Bachelor's degree, have completed specific nutrition/dietetics coursework, have supervised dietetics practice experience, and have passed a national exam. When you see an RD, it is important to find one who is experienced in diabetes care.

Nutrition education is a component of a comprehensive diabetes self-management education program. While making healthier food choices and understanding how different foods affect your blood glucose are something that all diabetes educators can help you with, RDs are the only members of the team who can provide medical nutrition therapy or more in-depth nutrition counseling.

RDs can help you learn to do the following:

- Plan meals to meet your nutrition needs

- Decipher food labels and understand key ingredients

- "Lighten up" your favorite recipes

- Modify diabetes meal plans to meet additional nutrition needs

- Include foods you enjoy in your meal plan

- Balance food and activity with your medication

When is it especially beneficial for you to see an RD? If you have diabetes complications such as kidney disease, digestive problems, or heart disease, dietitians can address your more complex nutrition needs. And if you have other unique nutrition issues not specific to diabetes—such as food allergies or intolerance, sports competition training, or preparations for gastric bypass surgery—RDs can also help.

 FOR YOUR SAFETY

In most areas of the United States, anyone can call themselves a nutritionist without actual qualifications. Use of RD and RDN is legally protected and can only be used by health-care professionals who meet the criteria to hold those credentials. Therefore, to assure you are getting sound nutrition advice from a qualified professional, look for the RD or RDN credential.

Other Team Members

Because diabetes can lead to other health complications, it helps to be proactive in all areas of your health. Having regular exams can help prevent problems or catch them in very early stages, when treatment is easier. Therefore, the following are some additional health-care professionals who don't specialize in diabetes but can or should still be included on your diabetes care team.

Eye doctor: Because eye damage is much more treatable when discovered early, we recommend having an eye doctor (either an ophthalmologist or optometrist) on your team. Annual exams with your eye doctor can catch any changes in your sight and general eye health from year to year. Ask your eye doctor about experience with patients who have diabetes and understanding treatment options.

Dentist: When you have diabetes, you are more likely to get gum disease. This is especially true if your blood glucose has been elevated. Therefore, it's important to let your dentist know you have diabetes and to visit the dentist's office every six months to help decrease the risk of gum disease and tooth loss. Brushing your teeth twice a day and flossing daily can also go a long way to preventing tooth decay and gum disease.

Podiatrist: Nerve damage and circulation issues caused by diabetes can lead to problems with your feet. Numbness and decreased blood flow can increase the risk of sores and infection. Even something that looks like a simple callus might be hiding a bigger problem underneath. It is important for you to look at your own feet daily to check for any redness, swelling, cuts, blisters, or cracks in the skin of your feet that could be signs of larger issues. Contact your medical provider if you see anything suspicious. Your medical provider can determine the need for a referral to a podiatrist. Podiatrists have specialized training to treat these type of foot problems.

Pharmacist: Pharmacists are medication experts, making them helpful to talk to about any diabetes medications you're taking. Some of the things a pharmacist can do for you are: identify potential drug interactions, counsel you on how medications work, recommend over-the-counter medications (taking into account your prescription medications and medical condition), and advise you about potential medication side effects. Pharmacists must be licensed in their state of employment. Credentials for pharmacists include RPh and PharmD.

Psychologist or counselor: Diabetes can contribute to so many different emotions, including anxiety and depression. Your feelings can also be all over the map when you're making changes to your life to manage your diabetes. If you feel you need help dealing with your emotions, you can add a psychologist or counselor to your team. Counselors may be licensed clinical social workers or other qualified health-care professionals, while psychologists may hold a doctorate degree or a Master's degree in psychology. To get in touch with one, your primary care provider will need to make a referral for you. Not all clinical psychologists or counselors accept insurance, so you will want to check on that before your first visit.

Physical therapist: If you're having difficulty getting started with regular physical activity, your primary care provider can refer you to a physical therapist. Even if you're dealing with limitations due to diabetes complications or other physical issues, exercise is beneficial for your overall health. A physical therapist can evaluate you and help you come up with an activity plan while improving your physical ability to exercise. Even if you've suffered from an injury or had surgery, a physical therapist can work with you to regain strength and improve your activity level. Exercise physiologists and physical therapists can coordinate with your primary care provider to put together the best care plan for you.

Gaining Support from Others

You have already learned how important medical support is for your diabetes management efforts; the next step is getting support from the people in your personal life. When you have diabetes, it is too difficult to go it alone performing your day-to-day activities. By enlisting support from your family, friends, and co-workers, you can get the help you need and reinforce the positive changes you are making.

However, it's not as simple as them being there—it's also about supporting you in the way you respond best. Apart from mind reading, they won't know how to do so unless you tell them. So how can you make sure they "get it" and give you the help you need? Read on to learn how!

Family

Family members are the people who love you no matter what. This makes them great allies—and also the people who are the easiest on which to take out your anger, frustration, disappointment, or other negative behaviors. That's why when family members offer support for your diabetes management in an unwanted way, it is easy to respond with strong emotions that wouldn't be displayed to strangers.

 DIABETES DECODED

Invite someone to officially be your "diabetes support person." The role of a diabetes support person is to help you with your efforts to successfully manage your diabetes. You can certainly have more than one! They could be co-workers, friends, family members, or anyone you talk with on a regular basis.

For example, one of the ways family members can offer unwanted support is by telling or "reminding" you that you can't eat something with comments like, "Are you supposed to be eating that cake? You're not supposed to eat cake. You had better stop eating that." It's like having the food police living with you! In return, you might respond, "Quit telling me what I can't eat," followed by thoughts such as *I'll show her, I'm going to eat twice as much now*. Hardly anyone's natural reaction would be to be grateful for this reminder and say "Oh, thank you very much for the reminder. I wouldn't have thought of that on my own." (Well, maybe with a very sarcastic tone someone might.)

Luckily, there is a communication tool you can use that can be very helpful in situations where your family members aren't providing the support you desire. You can break down your words as follows:

1. **Describe:** "When you _____"

2. **Explain:** "I feel _____"

3. **Specify:** "If you would do _____ instead"

4. **Consequence:** "I will feel _____"

Here's how this would look using the cake example:

1. **Describe:** "When you tell me I can't eat cake"

2. **Explain:** "It makes me feel like I want to eat more cake"

3. **Specify:** "If you would go for a walk with me instead"

4. **Consequence:** "I will feel that you are supporting me"

It is a good idea to practice this a few times before you try it out on someone else, so it feels more natural. You can then think of things your family members can do to support you. It's important to be specific about what it is you want. If you stop at telling them what it is you *don't* want them to do, they will flounder and probably do the same thing again. Once you let them know what specifically they can do, you will both benefit.

Another way your family can support you is by attending diabetes education classes with you. They can learn along with you that there are ways for you to have your cake and eat it, too!

Friends and Co-Workers

Friends and co-workers can provide a great opportunity for additional support for your diabetes management. Friends are a little more like family, so like family, it is a good idea to tell them specifically how they can support you. For instance, if you and your friends usually go out for pizza on Friday nights and you decide it's too difficult not to overeat, let them know. You can even offer an alternative, like taking turns preparing healthy recipes or choosing a new restaurant that makes it easier for you to stay on track.

As for support from your co-workers, many larger companies offer worksite wellness programs, walking clubs, or weight management programs. By participating in these programs, you may find that a number of your co-workers have similar fitness and even diabetes goals. Even if these programs aren't offered at your workplace, you can still invite co-workers to start walking with you at lunch time or make a pact with a co-worker to bring fruit and vegetables to replace the high-calorie snack options that take up residence in the break room.

The Least You Need to Know

- You need support to successfully manage your diabetes.
- With a diabetes care team, you can have health-care professionals experienced in diabetes care and management, as well as other areas of your health that can be affected by diabetes.
- Support from family and friends is important to stay on track. Improving communication and being specific with requests for help can minimize your frustration and maximize results.

Avoiding Short- and Long-Term Diabetes Complications

Now that you've put together your diabetes care team and put yourself in the right frame of mind for change, it's time to learn what you'll need to be aware of concerning your blood glucose. Diabetes can unfortunately lead to problems with your eyes, kidneys, heart, nerves, and blood vessels, especially when your blood glucose stays above target over a long period of time. Therefore, keeping your blood glucose in a recommended range helps decrease the likelihood of developing complications of diabetes.

This chapter discusses how to reduce risk of both short-term and long-term diabetes complications and identifies when you should seek help from others.

In This Chapter

- The target blood glucose range
- Hypoglycemia and hyperglycemia prevention and treatment strategies
- How others can help you
- Potential long-term complications of high blood glucose

Aiming for Your Target Blood Glucose

Things start to go wrong with your health when your blood glucose either stays too high (hyperglycemia) or goes too low (hypoglycemia). The problems caused by hyperglycemia generally develop slowly over time, although hyperglycemia can result in a medical emergency more quickly for people with type 1 diabetes, people with type 2 diabetes who are no longer making sufficient insulin, and older adults with diabetes. On the other hand, hypoglycemia is an urgent situation that requires an immediate response and, when severe, assistance from others for treatment. Therefore, knowing your target blood glucose range is the first step in helping you stay on track with your diabetes self-care. Blood glucose management targets are set at levels that help minimize the risk of diabetes complications. The ADA recommends the following blood glucose targets (measurements are explained in Chapter 1):

- **Fasting and before meals:** 80 to 130 mg/dL

- **One to two hours after the beginning of a meal:** Less than 180 mg/dL

Even though these are recommended numbers, when it comes to the target range for fasting and before meals, the high and low end may not work for everyone. For safety, many people with diabetes aim for a more practical target blood glucose of 100 mg/dL.

So what issues can arise at each end of the target range? For instance, the low end of the target range may be too low for people at risk for severe hypoglycemia. Higher blood glucose targets may be recommended with one or more of the following conditions:

- *Hypoglycemia unawareness*

- Frequent low blood glucose episodes

- Older adult with other complex health conditions

- Advanced heart disease or other advanced diabetes complications

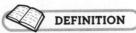 **DEFINITION**

> **Hypoglycemia unawareness** happens when a person with diabetes doesn't feel the early warning signs of low blood glucose, such as being dizzy, shaky, hungry, or irritable. People with hypoglycemia unawareness are more likely to experience severe consequences like stupor, seizures, or loss of consciousness without warning. This condition is more common in people with a history of chronic hypoglycemia, such as those with longstanding type 1 diabetes or those with type 2 diabetes who are taking certain diabetes medications (including insulin) that can contribute to low blood sugar.

Just as with the low end of the target being too low for some, it may also be appropriate to have an upper range that differs from the recommended maximum. An example of when blood glucose targets are set lower than usual is during pregnancy. Women with gestational diabetes, or those who have pre-existing diabetes and are pregnant, need to have their blood glucose in very good control for the best pregnancy outcome. In fact, it is recommended that women with diabetes who are considering pregnancy should take action to have blood glucose near normal prior to becoming pregnant. If this applies to you, make an appointment right away to see your medical provider to develop a plan.

As you can see, one size does not fit all when it comes to blood glucose. Therefore, it is best to work with your diabetes care team to establish individualized guidelines based on your medical needs and lifestyle.

How Low Is Too Low?

Blood glucose at or below 70 mg/dL is generally considered hypoglycemia, also referred to as hypo, low, low blood sugar reaction, or (when severe) insulin shock. This happens when the insulin level in your blood is elevated, causing the glucose in your blood to go too low. Hypoglycemia is considered a short-term diabetes complication because it occurs suddenly and is resolved quickly when appropriately treated.

Certain diabetes medications and insulin increase the risk for hypoglycemia. If your blood glucose is near normal, low blood glucose may occur more frequently. Other contributors to low blood sugar include not eating enough for the amount of medication taken, missing a meal or not eating on time, more physical activity than usual, and drinking alcohol without eating.

Ways to Prevent Hypoglycemia

It is better to prevent hypoglycemia in the first place than to have to treat low blood glucose. Here are some steps you can take to prevent hypoglycemia:

- Carry a snack with you in case of a delayed meal.

- Take your medication and/or insulin on time.

- Eat the right amount of food for your medication and/or insulin, or ask your medical provider about learning how to self-adjust your insulin based on your food intake.

- Check with your medical provider before drinking alcohol. Don't drink alcohol unless you are eating (see Chapter 8 for more on alcohol intake).

- Plan your physical activity around your meal schedule. If you are exercising more than an hour, you may need an extra snack. However, a snack is usually not needed if your activity is less than an hour.

- Carry fast-acting carbohydrates and a snack with you when you exercise.

 FOR YOUR SAFETY

Even with the best plans, hypoglycemia may still occur. Therefore, it is a good idea to wear or carry some form of medical identification, so in case of an emergency, others will know you have diabetes. It is especially important to wear a medical identification bracelet or necklace if you use insulin or take diabetes medication. Diabetes identification wallet cards are also available if you don't take any medicine for diabetes. Ask your medical provider or diabetes educator to find out more.

You can make it easier to follow these steps by establishing a meal and medication schedule. Not only will this help you on your typical days, it also will help prepare you for days that are not as predictable. For instance, if you usually eat dinner at 6:00 P.M. but it is going to be delayed until 8:00 P.M., you should plan to eat a snack by 6:00 P.M. to keep your blood sugar from going too low. Don't overdo it with the snack though, or you'll end up with a high blood glucose result before your 8:00 P.M. dinner. Check out Part 5 for more on diabetes meal planning.

Treating Hypoglycemia

The only way you can be sure your blood glucose is low is to test it. If you're not able to test but you feel like you're blood sugar is low, don't wait—treat it. Recognizing hypoglycemia and treating it early will help prevent it from becoming severe and turning into a medical emergency. Signs and symptoms of hypoglycemia are when you feel the following:

- Nervous or anxious

- Light headed or dizzy

- Shaky

- Sweaty

- Irritable

- Hungry

- Rapid heartbeat

- Numbness or tingling of your mouth or lips

If you experience these symptoms, check your blood sugar. If it is at or below 70 mg/dL, use the "15-15 rule" as a way to remember the steps to bring your blood glucose back into the target range:

1. Consume 15 g of carbohydrate, such as 3 to 4 glucose tablets, 4 ounces of fruit juice, 4 ounces of regular (not diet) soda, 15 small or 6 regular-size jelly beans, or 3 to 4 hard candies.

2. Wait 15 minutes and then check your blood glucose again.

If after the 15 minutes your blood sugar is still below 70 mg/dL, repeat the steps. If it is above 70 mg/dL, eat a meal or a snack within an hour to prevent your blood glucose from going too low again.

While anyone can have a low blood glucose reaction, if you take diabetes medication or insulin, you are at a higher risk. Therefore, always carry a source of fast-acting carbohydrate with you to help you stay prepared in case you need to treat hypoglycemia. The best treatment for low blood sugar is glucose. Glucose is available in tablet, gel, and liquid form at any drug store or grocery store pharmacy section. Glucose sources are easy to carry and have a long shelf life. Any fast-acting carbohydrate, like a candy that is primarily just sugar (such as jelly beans or gummy bears), also works. While soft candy is easier to eat when experiencing hypoglycemic symptoms, hard candy is often more readily available. It is not recommended you use chocolate or candy bars to treat hypoglycemia because they contain fat and are not as quick or effective in raising the blood glucose as the other pure carbohydrate sources we've mentioned.

 FOR YOUR SAFETY

Try not to overtreat low blood sugar. Experiencing hypoglycemia is very uncomfortable, to say the least; it is easy to feel like you want to eat everything in sight to make the symptoms go away. Instead, try to stay calm and follow the 15-15 rule. Eating too much can cause a high blood glucose that may be difficult to correct.

How Others Can Help You Treat Hypoglycemia

It is a good idea to share the information about symptoms and treatment of hypoglycemia with the people close to you. That way, they can be aware of potential issues that could come up. Once familiar with your symptoms, others may actually recognize your low blood glucose even before you do.

While treating hypoglycemia early on your own is best, you may need assistance from others at some point; therefore, review with them how they can help when you have hypoglycemia. Make sure others understand what you need when your blood sugar is low. For instance, a well-meaning person may offer you a diet soda instead of regular soda because she doesn't understand that at that moment what you really need is sugar. Also, make sure people close to you know not to try to have you swallow something if you lose consciousness; it could cause you to choke.

You generally need assistance from others if the following symptoms of hypoglycemia occur:

- Poor coordination
- Slurred speech
- Difficulty concentrating
- Blurry vision
- Feeling weak or tired

These more serious symptoms can set in when your brain is not getting enough glucose for fuel. As long as you are conscious and can follow commands, others can help you eat or drink glucose sources that are easy to swallow, such as apple juice or glucose gel.

 FOR YOUR SAFETY

Call your medical provider if you have had several episodes of hypoglycemia, especially if you can't figure out why. There are many factors that contribute to hypoglycemia, so make sure to let your provider know the circumstances at the time of the episodes.

When Is Hypoglycemia an Emergency?

Hypoglycemia is a medical emergency if your blood glucose goes so low that you lose consciousness and pass out. Though this is uncommon, if it occurs, you are totally dependent on others. Someone you are close to needs to know what to do in this situation. Also, ask your medical provider if you should be prescribed glucagon. Glucagon is given as an injection by someone else and acts to raise your blood glucose and help you regain consciousness. It is recommended that a health-care professional review the instructions on how to give the shot with the person you choose, in case you ever need it. If given, you should be rolled onto your side to prevent choking, as glucagon may cause vomiting.

To be safe, it is best to have your diabetes support person (or people) know that 911 should be called if you ever pass out. Even if glucagon is available, additional monitoring by emergency response services (EMS) is beneficial, especially if a complication should arise. EMS professionals are trained to respond to hypoglycemia on site, with transport to the emergency room when necessary.

How High Is Too High?

Symptoms of hyperglycemia generally develop when the blood glucose is elevated above 200 mg/dL. The symptoms of hyperglycemia are the same as those that may present when your diabetes is first diagnosed (covered in Chapters 1 and 2). However, these symptoms may not be obvious for days or even weeks, so you can't really go by how you feel to discover and treat high blood glucose. Still, there are a number of things that can contribute to hyperglycemia, including the following:

- Overeating, especially high-carbohydrate foods

- Taking too little diabetes medication and/or insulin

- Using the incorrect technique to inject insulin

- Using expired diabetes medications or insulin

- Taking medications that raise the blood glucose, such as steroids

- Surgery, illness, or infection

- Increased emotional stress

The longer your blood glucose stays elevated, the worse things get. When your blood glucose is very elevated, it can lead to a condition called *glucose toxicity*. If left untreated, eventually the beta cells of the pancreas are no longer able to secrete insulin.

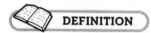 **DEFINITION**

> **Glucose toxicity** is a "vicious cycle" in which hyperglycemia itself contributes to even higher blood glucose levels. The hyperglycemia causes injury to the beta cells of the pancreas, causing less insulin production and then more insulin resistance. The good news is that it is reversible by getting the blood glucose levels under control.

Treating Hyperglycemia

If you have type 2 diabetes and your blood glucose is elevated, a simple thing to start with is to drink a few glasses of water and take a walk. If your blood glucose has been elevated for some time, you may be a bit dehydrated due to increased urination. While drinking water alone won't lower your blood glucose, dehydration makes matters worse. Taking a walk or similar physical activity lowers blood glucose by stimulating muscle cells to take up glucose better and improving insulin sensitivity. (You'll learn more about physical activity to manage your health in Chapter 7.) For type 2 diabetes, insulin injections are also sometimes used short term to break a cycle of hyperglycemia.

Taking corrective action based on blood glucose monitoring results will help you avoid problems caused by hyperglycemia. (More information on blood glucose meters, how to test, and how to keep your blood glucose in the target range is discussed in Chapter 11.) If you've tried the previous suggestions to lower your blood glucose, it is important to follow up with additional blood glucose testing to see if your actions corrected the problem. If your blood glucose is at or above 250 mg/dL, check your blood glucose every four hours. If your blood glucose stays above 250 mg/dL for more than 24 hours or if your blood glucose goes above 400 mg/dL even one time, call your medical provider. If your blood glucose is high often, you may need to talk with your medical provider about a change in medication. Because food makes blood glucose go up, especially foods containing carbohydrates, you may also need to change how you're eating. (There is much more information on nutrition in Part 4 of this book.)

 DID YOU KNOW?

People with type 1 diabetes need to take action to lower blood glucose more quickly if ketones are present. When blood glucose is 250 mg/dL or higher, the urine should be tested for ketones. If ketones are present, insulin is generally needed to correct the situation. While it may seem like exercising would be a good solution to bring down blood glucose, that's not true when ketones are present. Exercise can actually make the blood glucose go higher, so it should be delayed until the blood glucose improves and the urine tests negative for ketones.

When Is Hyperglycemia an Emergency?

There are several types of life-threatening medical emergencies caused by hyperglycemia. While people with type 1 diabetes are more likely to develop DKA, it can also be seen in people with type 2 diabetes if they have become insulin deficient (DKA is discussed in Chapter 2). A condition called *hyperosmolor hyperglycemic state (HHS)* also occurs in people with type 2 diabetes, especially older adults. HHS is triggered by extreme dehydration, which leads to blood glucose levels above 600 mg/dL without ketones.

You should also call your medical provider if you have any of the following symptoms:

- Vomiting or diarrhea for more than six hours, even if you're able to take in some food and fluid

- Fever over 101.5°F

- Signs of dehydration, such as sticky mouth and tongue, dry or cracked lips, or dark urine

You should call 911 if you have any of the following issues:

- Trouble breathing

- Shallow breathing, with a fruity odor to the breath

- Chest pain

Illness can also contribute to elevated blood glucose. So when you're sick, monitor your blood glucose frequently. Because it is common to need more diabetes medication or insulin when you're ill, don't stop taking your diabetes medication just because you're not eating as much as usual. It's also important to keep up with your fluid intake to help prevent dehydration and hyperglycemic emergencies. Call your medical provider if you have any questions about what to do during illness.

Long-Term Diabetes Complications

Untreated hyperglycemia can potentially lead to *long-term diabetes complications,* otherwise known as "chronic" complications. This happens when your blood glucose stays above target, but not high enough to lead to a medical emergency. Because the development of these complications is gradual, you may not be aware of what's happening. In the early stages of type 2 diabetes, you may feel fine even if your blood sugars are running high. But problems can still be developing.

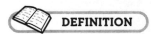 **DEFINITION**

> **Long-term diabetes complications** occur gradually when blood glucose has not been well managed over a period of years. The extra glucose traveling in the blood causes damage to both small and large blood vessels, as well as the nerves. Examples of long-term complications include blindness (damage to the retina in the eye), kidney failure, heart disease, and neuropathy (nerve damage causing numbness, tingling, and pain in the feet).

The end results of untreated hyperglycemia can be debilitating and even life-threatening. You may know someone who has become blind, started dialysis, suffered from a stroke, or had an amputation because of diabetes. However, with good blood glucose management, long-term diabetes complications aren't inevitable. Even if you have some of the symptoms of long-term diabetes complications that follow, getting your blood glucose in better control now may help prevent complications from getting worse. And if caught early enough, achieving blood glucose control can improve some symptoms, so don't give up.

Eye Problems

Diabetic retinopathy is a *microvascular complication* of diabetes that can lead to blindness. There is a strong link between hyperglycemia and the development of this complication, as elevated blood glucose causes damage to the tiny blood vessels of the retina in the back of the eye. Initially the blood vessels become swollen and then blocked, causing the retina to not receive enough nourishment. Eventually the retina is no longer receiving the blood supply it needs and new, weaker blood vessels begin to grow. These new blood vessels unfortunately are ineffective; the thin walls can easily break and blood can leak into the eye, leading to vision loss.

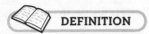 **DEFINITION**

Microvascular complication is a long-term complication of diabetes that damages the small blood vessels of the body. The commonly recognized microvascular complications include retinopathy (eyes), nephropathy (kidneys), and neuropathy (nerves).

Sometimes, your vision may get blurry when your blood glucose is elevated and slightly worsen as your blood glucose improves. However, this is not the same as diabetic retinopathy; it generally resolves when you achieve blood glucose control. Therefore, you shouldn't go out and get new glasses until after your blood glucose is in target for a few months because your vision may continue to change. You don't want to get stuck with an expensive pair of glasses you can't see out of. If necessary, you can use inexpensive reading glasses to tide you over.

Kidney Disease

Diabetes is the leading cause of kidney disease in the United States; kidney disease caused by diabetes is called *diabetic nephropathy*. In healthy kidneys, tiny parts of your kidneys known as nephrons filter your blood, eliminate waste products, and control fluid levels in the body. With diabetes, the nephrons slowly thicken, and scar tissue builds up. Hyperglycemia and high blood pressure can worsen the problem, and over time, the kidneys leak the protein albumin into your urine.

To detect early kidney disease, your medical provider can give you a simple urine test called a microalbumin test, which measures the amount of albumin in your urine. You can also slow the progression of kidney disease by quitting smoking if you smoke and keeping your blood pressure and blood glucose in control.

Nerve Damage

Diabetic neuropathy, or nerve damage caused by diabetes, can affect a number of body systems, including your urinary tract, your hands and feet, your digestive system, and even your heart. The most familiar complication is nerve damage that causes numbness and tingling in your feet, known as peripheral neuropathy. Symptoms of peripheral neuropathy occur first in the feet and then progress up the leg. The presentation can vary from person to person, but it has been described as sharp, stabbing pain; extreme sensitivity to touch; numbness; tingling; and pain when walking. Peripheral neuropathy can lead to foot ulcers, bone deformities, and joint pain. Your hands and arms can also be affected by neuropathy.

To be proactive against these issues, regular foot exams with your medical provider can help you spot issues before they turn into big problems. Take off your socks and shoes at each visit with your medical provider as a reminder to have her check your feet.

Macrovascular Complications

Heart disease, stroke, and peripheral artery disease are the *macrovascular complications* of diabetes, caused by large blood vessel damage. Factors increasing the risk of macrovascular complications include high blood glucose, high blood pressure, smoking, and high cholesterol. With type 2 diabetes, you often have high blood pressure, high "bad" cholesterol, low "good" cholesterol, and high triglycerides, all of which increase the risk of heart attack and stroke. Peripheral artery disease can lead to pain and poor circulation in the feet and increases the risk of amputation.

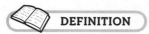 **DEFINITION**

> A **macrovascular complication** is a long-term complication of diabetes that affects the large blood vessels in the body, which leads to damage of the heart and brain.

Managing diabetes well and keeping blood pressure and cholesterol under control can help decrease your risk of macrovascular complications. Eating more healthfully, adding physical activity into your regular routine, and managing stress can also go a long way to improving your heart health and minimize your risk of complications (see Part 3 for more on diabetes management strategies).

The Least You Need to Know

- When blood glucose goes too high or too low, problems can occur. Therefore, blood glucose targets are set to decrease the risk of diabetes complications. Blood glucose monitoring can let you know if you are out of the target range and need to take corrective action.

- If you find your blood glucose is below 70 mg/dL, try the 15-15 rule: consume 15 g of carbohydrate, wait 15 minutes, and check your blood glucose again.

- While issues related to hyperglycemia aren't as immediately harmful as hypoglycemia, you can potentially develop life-threatening problems.

- High blood glucose over a long period of time can eventually lead to long-term diabetes complications, such as eye problems, kidney disease, nerve damage, and cardiovascular disease.

Diabetes Management Strategies

Now that you have built up your support network and are in the frame of mind to overcome your diabetes, it's time for us to provide you with tools for managing your diabetes. This part begins with how being physically active is one of the best things you can do for yourself when you have diabetes. You learn how to start moving, increase your activity throughout the day, and build up your strength via resistance training.

This part also discusses behaviors you can alter to better control your blood glucose, such as getting a good night's sleep, managing your stress levels, adjusting your alcohol intake, and quitting smoking. We even go over how supplements fit into the mix.

Beyond exercise and other behavioral changes, you can keep your blood glucose in control with diabetes pills, noninsulin injectable medications, and insulin as needed. So this part breaks down how diabetes medications and insulin work to improve blood glucose control, as well as the tools involved (such as insulin pens and pumps).

To track your progress, this part closes with information on monitoring your blood glucose with meters and even glucose sensors. You learn not only what the numbers mean, but what to do based on what you find out.

Get Moving

If there was something that could decrease your risk of heart disease, lower your blood pressure, improve your flexibility and balance, help you feel good about yourself, relieve your stress, get you to sleep better, burn calories to help you manage your weight, increase your energy level, and improve your quality of life, would you be interested? It sounds too good to be true, doesn't it? Well, guess what? There really is such a thing, and it doesn't have to cost you a dime. It's exercise!

Physical activity, along with a diabetes meal plan (see Part 5), is the cornerstone of therapy for diabetes self-management. This chapter discusses how physical activity helps you not only with diabetes management but overall health as well. We also go over activity guidelines for people with diabetes, as well as strategies for success when it comes to fitting physical activity into your usual routine. Now's the time to get moving!

In This Chapter

- How physical activity impacts blood glucose
- Aerobic activity and resistance training
- Tips for safe exercise
- Getting started if you're new to physical activity

Physical Activity—Insulin's Helper

While physical activity has multiple benefits for just about everyone, when you have diabetes, physical activity can be especially helpful in controlling your blood glucose. That's because when you're active, your cells become more sensitive to insulin. Insulin you take or insulin your body is making then works more efficiently to help get glucose out of your blood and into your cells, where you use it as energy.

Insulin resistance—the term used when your body isn't using insulin well—can be significantly decreased with physical activity. If you're insulin resistant and therefore need more insulin to get the same blood glucose–lowering effect as people who aren't insulin resistant, it can be more difficult for you to lose or maintain weight. Regular physical activity not only helps you burn more calories, it can also lower the amount of insulin or diabetes medications you need to achieve your target blood glucose levels. Burning off extra calories and being able to use less insulin for blood glucose control are beneficial for weight management.

So how does all of this work? Your body breaks down carbohydrates from the food you eat into glucose for fuel or energy. Because you don't eat 24/7, your body also stores glucose for use later when you're not eating. When the glucose is put into storage, it is formed into another type of sugar called *glycogen*. You can then tap into those sugar stores for extra fuel when needed; when your blood glucose is lower, the glycogen is converted back into glucose for use.

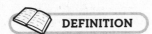 **DEFINITION**

> **Glycogen** is the main source of stored carbohydrates in the body. When glucose is
> not needed for energy, it is converted to glycogen and stored mainly in the liver and
> muscles.

One of the places your body stores glycogen is your muscle cells. During physical activity, your muscles burn the stored glycogen. Afterward, your muscles use glucose from your blood to replace the glycogen that was used, so you end up with lower blood sugar levels. Plus, the contraction of your muscle cells provides a separate mechanism that helps control your blood glucose. When your muscle cells contract, they can take up glucose more efficiently even without insulin's help. With regular physical activity, you can improve your muscles' ability to use this mechanism—the more you exercise, the better this works.

Therefore, to maintain improved blood glucose control, plan on regular physical activity at least every other day. If you can do more, that's even better. Even shorter bursts of activity help. You can improve insulin sensitivity for up to several days with activities that last longer and make you work harder.

Aerobic Exercise

The word *aerobics* may conjure up an image of a room with an instructor smiling and shouting out directions to a group of people sweating to energizing music. However, the word *aerobic* simply means "oxygen requiring." So in addition to taking an aerobics class, some examples of aerobic exercises are brisk walking, riding a bike, swimming, dancing, skating, skiing, and jogging. If you mow the lawn, vacuum, rake leaves, or climb up and down the stairs with laundry, those household chores count, too. Moving the large muscles in your legs, getting your heart rate up, breaking a sweat, and breathing a bit harder are signs of moderate aerobic activity.

Because aerobic activities burn more calories and are more effective at lowering blood glucose than strength training, it is recommended that people with diabetes include moderate aerobic activity 150 minutes a week. You should spread the exercise throughout the week, exercising on most days and not going more than two days without physical activity. You can also think of that as 30 minutes of activity 5 days a week if that works for you. However, if you are just starting out, 10 minutes a day is okay. After all, adding 10 minutes of activity to your day is 10 minutes more than you were doing! You can then gradually work to increase your activity level at your own pace.

 DIABETES DECODED

Picking a fun leisure activity will help you with your fitness goal. Have you ever wanted to try salsa dancing? Did you used to bowl but haven't picked up a ball in a while? Would you like to take a swing at golf? Think of something you would enjoy and try it. Make it something your whole family would enjoy to help them get fit as well!

To really have a good shot at maintaining an exercise routine, it helps if you choose something you like to do. If you hate jogging but enjoy walking your dog around the neighborhood, walk the dog. You can burn the same amount of calories; you just have to walk for a longer amount of time, compared to if you were jogging, to accomplish it.

Resistance Training

Weight gain generally happens as people age due to a slowing metabolism due to decreased muscle mass and a more sedentary lifestyle, among other factors. If you don't do anything about it, your muscles will begin to start shrinking and wasting away somewhere after age 40. You can lose about 8 percent of your muscle mass between ages 40 and 50, and that speeds up to an approximately 15 percent loss per decade after age 75. While you can't totally eliminate this process, you can fight back by staying active. Want to hear some great news? You can build muscle at any age! That's right, building muscle is not just for teenagers and young adults.

Resistance training, also called *strength training,* is most helpful for maintaining muscle mass. The more muscle mass you keep, the better your metabolism, because more muscle helps you burn more calories, meaning you're less likely to gain weight. You can also increase the amount of muscle you currently have. Studies have shown that even older adults ages 70 and above can improve muscle mass using resistance training.

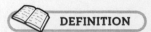 **DEFINITION**

> **Resistance training** is using exercise that causes the muscles to contract against an external resistance (which can be your own body weight, dumbbells, stretch bands, cans, or other items that cause your muscles to contract). This type of training improves strength, tone, the size of muscles, or endurance.

The goal of resistance training is not to turn you into a body builder with bulging biceps; rather, it is to increase your strength, function, and balance. Everyday activities can become easier with resistance training. For example, when you get up from a low sofa, do you have to use your hands to push yourself up? After performing some strengthening resistance exercises over time, you might just be able to get up from that couch without using your hands, because you've built up the muscles in your thighs and stomach that help you get up and down more easily.

Resistance training exercises using hand weights (even soup cans to start), elastic bands, or gym weight machines can all help you build muscle. Using your own body weight for resistance counts, too. Aim for some resistance training two to three days a week, with 10 to 15 repetitions for each exercise. You can then gradually work up to three sets of 10 to 15 of each exercise, three days a week.

Not sure where to begin? The following are a couple simple exercises to start with. Remember, first talk with your medical provider about any restrictions or limitations you might have, and read through all the steps carefully before starting.

Wall Push-Up

If you're unable to complete a regular push-up, try this modified version; this easier alternative won't strain your back. Once you build up your muscle strength, you can progress to a more challenging version using a countertop, bench, or sturdy chair instead of the wall.

1. Stand a little farther than arm's length away from a wall. Set your feet about the same width as your shoulders.

2. Lean your body forward and put your palms flat against the wall at shoulder height and shoulder-width apart. Slowly breathe in as you bend your elbows and lower your upper body toward the wall. Do this as a slow, controlled motion while keeping your feet flat on the floor. Hold the position with your elbows bent for one second.

3. Breathe out and slowly push yourself back until your arms are straight.

4. Repeat 10 to 15 times, and then rest. If you can, repeat 10 to 15 more times.

Chair Stand

Do you want to be able to get up from the sofa easier? How about in and out of the car? Here is an exercise to help build up those muscles.

1. Sit up straight toward the front of a sturdy chair, knees bent. Place your feet flat on floor, shoulder-width apart.

2. Lean slightly back (without touching the back of the chair) with your hands crossed over your chest, keeping your back and shoulders straight throughout. Breathe in slowly.

3. Breathe out and bring your upper body forward until you're sitting upright again.

4. Extend your arms out in front of you, parallel to the floor, and slowly stand up.

5. Breathe in as you slowly sit down.

6. Repeat 10 to 15 times, and then rest. If you can, repeat 10 to 15 more times.

Checking Your Exercise Intensity

In order to get the most benefit from physical activity, you should aim for moderate intensity. How do you know you're doing physical activity at a moderate intensity level? For most people with type 2 diabetes, an example of moderate activity is walking at a brisk pace. However, it can vary from person to person based on how fit you are. Moderate activity takes some effort and should feel a bit difficult. For instance, you're breathing more quickly but not out of breath, and after approximately 10 minutes, you start breaking a sweat.

While this gives you a general idea of what moderate activity feels like, the following are a couple ways to more specifically gauge your own exercise intensity.

Measuring Your Heart Rate

One way you can figure out if you are exercising with moderate intensity is by measuring your heart rate. By counting your heartbeats during exercise, you can tell how hard your heart is working. To use your target heart rate to measure exercise intensity, you need to know what your maximum heart rate is first. This is the maximum that your heart should beat in one minute while you're exercising.

FOR YOUR SAFETY

Keep in mind that the target heart rate calculation is for a general range based on your age. Because certain medications and medical conditions can affect your heart rate, your target may be different than what is listed here. Talk with your medical provider to see what's right for you.

The following shows you how to find your maximum heart rate:

220 – your age = maximum heart rate

So, for example, if you are 30 years old, you subtract 30 from 220:

220 – 30 = 190

As you can see, if you're 30 years old, your maximum heart rate is 190 beats per minute. Once you have this number, you can calculate your target rate. Moderate intensity is generally a target of 50 to 70 percent of your maximum heart rate (if you are less fit, you may want to aim for the lower part of the target):

maximum heart rate × .5 = target heart rate (low end)

maximum heart rate × .7 = target heart rate (high end)

Continuing with the previous example, if 190 is your maximum heart rate, you would multiply that by .5 and .7 to get your target heart rate:

190 × .5 = 95

190 × .7 = 133

In this example, your target heart rate would be 95 to 133 beats per minute. This is referred to as a target heart rate zone.

Now that you know your target heart rate zone, it's time to find your pulse. There are two places you can use: your neck and your wrist. You can find your carotid pulse by placing your index and third fingers on your neck to the side of your windpipe. If you'd rather use your wrist (radial artery), place two fingers between the bone and the tendon on the thumb side of your wrist. Once you've located and placed your fingers on the area of your choosing, count the heartbeats for 15 seconds and multiply by 4 to get the number of beats per minute. You can try this before you start your activity to get your resting heart rate. For most adults, the resting heart rate is between 60 to 100 beats per minute.

Next time you exercise, you can check your pulse and then compare that number to your target rate zone to see if you're where you should be. If your heart rate is above the upper limit of your target heart rate zone, you need to slow down. If your target heart rate is below the target heart range, you can try exercising a bit harder. You want to be exercising enough to get the benefit but not overdoing it. Make sure to listen to the rest of your body as well; if you're short of breath you need to slow down.

If all of this sounds like too much to deal with, you can also use a heart rate monitor during exercise. This is also a good option if you'd like to know your numbers during exercise without stopping and checking your heart rate.

The Talk Test and Perceived Exertion

For most people, the talk test or perceived exertion work well to estimate exercise intensity. They are subjective measures that have to do with how you personally feel, rather than an objective measure like heart rate. The talk test is an easy way to determine your exercise intensity without stopping to check your heart rate. If you're exercising at a moderate intensity, you should be able to talk but not be able to sing. If you're walking along and you can carry on a conversation with your walking partner, that's a good thing. If you're walking along and you can sing or whistle, you can probably pick up the pace! If you're a little short of breath, that's okay; however, if you feel like you can't catch your breath, you need to slow down.

Perceived exertion, based on how you feel during a particular activity, is another way to determine how hard you're exercising. The Borg Rating of Perceived Exertion is a scale that can be used to rate how hard you feel your body is working during physical activity. Levels of perceived exertion are rated based on awareness of physical changes, such as increased heart rate, breathing rate, sweating, and muscle fatigue during exercise. The lowest number on the scale, 6, means "no exertion at all," while 20, the highest number on the scale, equals "maximal exertion." A rating of 12 to 14 ("somewhat hard") is a moderate level of exercise intensity. By becoming more in tune with the physical changes that happen during exercise, you'll know better when to pick up the pace or slow it down.

 DIABETES DECODED

For more information and specific instructions for the Borg Rating of Perceived Exertion scale, go to cdc.gov/physicalactivity/everyone/measuring/exertion.html.

Exercise Safety Tips

Before starting a new exercise routine, it's always a good idea to talk with your medical provider and ask about any safety precautions you need to follow. You may have restrictions you need to be aware of, especially if you have certain diabetes complications. Beyond that, the following are some things you should do or be aware of as you're ramping up your physical activity.

Watching Your Blood Sugar

Exercise can contribute to hypoglycemia, so always be prepared with a source of carbohydrates with you while exercising. Generally, if you are starting out with a walking program that is 30 minutes or less at a time, for example, you won't need adjustments to diabetes medication or insulin or need to add a snack. However, vigorous exercise or exercising for longer periods of time increases the risk. For insulin users, hypoglycemia may happen up to 24 hours after activity in those situations. If you're going to be exercising for over an hour, you will likely need to adjust your insulin or add in a snack containing carbohydrates. Talk with your provider about what's right for you. In case of low blood sugar, carry glucose tablets in your pocket—don't just leave them in your gym bag.

If hypoglycemia is a problem, monitoring your blood glucose more closely will help you come up with a solution. (See Chapter 6 for more information on treating low blood sugar.)

Avoiding Injury

You may have heard the line "no pain, no gain"; well that's definitely not true. You need to be cautious about pushing yourself too hard. If you feel too short of breath, more than just mild pain, or just can't finish your workout, you might be trying to do too much.

How difficult you perceive your exertion or exercise effort for a certain activity matters. It could be very different from what another person is experiencing doing the same thing. It depends on how much more or less fit they are then you. Don't compare yourself to someone else and push too hard to match what they do. Keep within the moderate pace, if you're new to exercise. As your fitness level improves, you will be able to push yourself more.

 FOR YOUR SAFETY

If you're not sure how to do an exercise, look for a demonstration of the proper way to complete it. That way, you can prevent any potential injuries from doing it incorrectly. If you are reading the steps to complete an exercise, read it thoroughly before starting. Using a video, pictures in a book, or working with a fitness specialist can all be beneficial. It's also a good idea to read the steps of the exercise thoroughly before starting to understand the motions.

However, no matter your fitness level, having a warm-up and cool down before moderate or vigorous activity is key to lessening your risk of injury. You can warm up with the same type of activity you will be using for your workout. For example, if you are planning to walk for 30 minutes, start out walking slowly for the first 5 minutes to warm up and gradually increase your heart rate.

When you've finished your exercise, your heart rate is higher, your body temperature is elevated, and your blood is flowing faster. If you stop exercising suddenly, you might not feel well and you could even pass out. Slowing down your pace for the last five minutes will help your heart rate and temperature return to pre-exercise levels. Because your muscles and joints are still warm after a workout, it's a good idea to include stretching in your cool down. Stretching can improve flexibility and help decrease muscle cramps. Stretches should be held for about 10 to 30 seconds and shouldn't be painful. Never bounce when stretching to avoid injury, and make sure to breathe!

Even a Little Bit Counts

Did all of this talk about working out at a moderate pace for five days a week overwhelm you? If you are a member of the couch potato club, don't despair; even a little bit of activity can help improve your fitness. The most important thing is getting started and then building it up. Even 10 minutes of activity holds some health benefits. As a matter of fact, the less fit you are, the more a little bit of activity does help. For example, a trained Olympic athlete is not going to see much if any benefit from 10 minutes of walking. But if you haven't been walking at all, that 10 minutes can make a difference. As your fitness level increases, you'll need to add in more activity.

Remember, when setting fitness goals (covered in Chapter 4), you also need to address barriers. Common reasons for not exercising are not having enough time, being too tired, having no one to exercise with, and bad weather. You not only have to plan how to add activity into your day, you also need to figure out how to break down those barriers! Just start where you can start.

Stepping Your Way to Success

One easy way to get yourself moving more is walking. After all, fitness goals can not only be counted in minutes and distance, but also by how many steps you take. You may have heard about the goal of getting 10,000 steps a day. While that is a wonderful goal, it may not be realistic for you. Just try to get moving more than you already are.

How can you find out? If you get a pedometer or other fitness tracker and wear it for a few days, you'll get a good idea of your baseline. Pedometers can be as simple as a "step counter" or more complex, measuring things such as distance in miles, calories burned, floors climbed, and so on. The least expensive pedometers cost around $5, while some fitness trackers with all the "bells and whistles" can cost hundreds of dollars. (If you'd like to compare, some of the more popular fitness trackers are listed in Appendix B.)

Whatever you decide upon to track your steps, start by not changing anything the first few days you wear it. Once you find out how many steps a day you take on average, you can then choose a goal that will work for you. For instance, if you walk about 2,000 steps a day, increasing your steps by 500 per day over the next two weeks may be reasonable. If you reach your goal sooner, set another one. Step it up!

> **DIABETES DECODED**
>
> If your sole reason for exercise is to lose weight without making any additional changes, you may need to re-evaluate. Physical activity helps with weight management and improves your fitness level while losing weight, but you still need to reduce the amount of calories you eat. So set yourself up for success by making manageable changes to eat healthier and to step up your activity at the same time.

Adding Activity in Your Day

If you're not ready yet to set an official exercise goal, you can simply add more exercise to activities you normally complete during the day. Here are some examples of things you can do to get moving:

- Park your car farther away when you go to work, the store, or are running errands.

- Take a lap around the outside perimeter of the grocery store before you start shopping. (Just walk quickly past the bakery department!)

- Take one flight of stairs before getting on the elevator. Better yet, walk up more flights.

- Walk up and down the stairs at home more. Don't pile things up on the bottom step to make less trips; make a separate trip for each item.

- Get up and walk around during TV commercials. Even getting up and down from your chair five times can help.

- Play a game of tag with your kids.

- Walk around when you talk on the phone.

- Stand up at least once every 30 minutes at work.

- Deliver a message to a co-worker in person rather than sending an email.

- Take a 10-minute walk on your lunch break.

- Walk the dog. If you don't have a dog, walk your neighbor's dog.

Pick one or two items from the list and start today! You know you can do it!

DID YOU KNOW?

The National Institute on Aging has a wonderful booklet complete with pictures of how to do some basic strengthening exercises called "Exercise and Physical Activity" that you can download free from their website at nia.nih.gov/health/publication/exercise. The website also has a link for the Go4Life program to help you increase your activity.

The Least You Need to Know

- Physical activity is important for diabetes management, as well as your overall health and wellness.
- Both aerobic activity and resistance training should be included in a regular exercise routine for people with diabetes.
- There are exercise safety precautions to be aware of when you have diabetes. For instance, exercise may cause low blood glucose or cause very high blood glucose to go higher.
- Additional physical activity can be incorporated into your everyday routine. Get up and move more often starting now!

Alcohol, Smoke, and Supplement Intake

While there are some behaviors known to increase your health risks, such as drinking alcohol and smoking tobacco, you may also be risking your health through actions you think you're taking to help it, such as consuming supplements. In this chapter, we go over how to safely fit alcohol into your diabetes plan, if you'd like to, as well as the importance of moderation. We then cover the ways smoking negatively affects your health, particularly with diabetes, and provide tips on how to quit. We close this chapter with a discussion on popular supplements that goes beyond the too-good-to-be-true claims with evidence of how they can (or can't) help you manage your diabetes.

In This Chapter

- The benefits and risks of drinking alcohol
- Why quitting smoking is important for your health
- Common dietary supplements and diabetes management

Consuming Alcohol

You may have heard that people with diabetes shouldn't drink alcohol. Have you wondered if that's really true? There are definitely some guidelines to follow when it comes to alcohol and diabetes. However, as it turns out, alcohol is not necessarily all bad.

 FOR YOUR SAFETY

Talk with your medical provider before you drink alcohol. Make sure your provider knows all the medications you are taking, including over-the-counter medications and supplements. Don't drink alcohol if you have a history of alcohol abuse or have a medical condition that worsens with alcohol consumption like cirrhosis. You should also avoid alcohol if you are pregnant or planning to become pregnant.

For most people with diabetes, a moderate amount of alcohol is okay. What does *moderate* mean? Moderate drinking is defined as having up to one drink a day for women or up to two drinks a day for men. One drink is equal to 12 ounces of beer, 5 ounces of wine, or 1.5 ounces of liquor. Along with these guidelines, it is recommended that neither men nor women have more than two drinks in a day. So, for example, you shouldn't "save up" by having nothing to drink during the week and then having a six-pack of beer on Saturday night.

The following table shows you common alcoholic drinks in the serving size that equals one drink according to the guidelines.

One-Drink Equivalent for Common Alcoholic Drinks

Beverage	Serving Size	Calories	Carbohydrates	Alcohol Content
Regular beer	12 oz.	145	13 g	14 g
Light beer	12 oz.	105	5 g	11 g
Red wine	5 oz.	125	4 g	16 g
White wine	5 oz.	122	4 g	15 g
Liquor (80-proof)	1.5 oz.	97	0 g	14 g

Data source: Calorieking.com

As you can see, the portion sizes can vary for the same amount of alcohol consumed. For example, if you've heard that beer or wine is safer to drink or doesn't have the same effect as liquor, that's not actually true; they just have a larger portion size for the same amount of alcohol content. While the amount of "pure" alcohol is the same in a serving of beer, wine, or liquor, the portion size is largest for beer because it has the lowest percentage of alcohol per volume. Therefore, if you drink the full 12 ounces of regular beer, you get the same amount of alcohol as in the 1.5 ounces of liquor.

Another consideration is the amount of calories and carbohydrates in the alcoholic drink you choose. All alcoholic drinks will increase your calorie intake, but some will more than others. The majority of calories in the drinks listed in the table come from the alcohol, with the remainder of the calories coming from carbohydrates. The light beer is lower in carbohydrates but not significantly lower in calories or alcohol. On the other hand, the hard liquor doesn't contain any carbohydrates, so all the calories are from the alcohol.

So is it okay for you to drink alcohol if you have diabetes? While there are some documented health benefits to alcohol, there are definitely health risks to it as well. Let's take a look at what those are.

Potential Risks from Alcohol

Anyone can experience short-term or long-term health risks with excessive or binge drinking. Binge drinking is considered four or more drinks in one sitting for women and five or more drinks in one sitting for men, while excessive drinking can be over a longer time period. Too much alcohol in the short term can affect judgment and lead to injuries, such as falls or car accidents. It can even cause alcohol poisoning, a medical emergency that's caused by a high level of alcohol in the blood.

 FOR YOUR SAFETY

You might have seen a label on one of your prescription bottles stating "Do not drink alcoholic beverages while taking this medication." With some medications, it may still be okay to drink in moderation even if this label is on the bottle; with others, it's not. How can you find out? Talk with the medical provider who prescribed the medication to ask what the specific precautions should be, including whether combining alcohol with your diabetes medication can make it more likely for you to have a low blood sugar reaction. Make sure to learn about any side effects of your medications and understand how alcohol might impact them.

Long-term health risks of excessive alcohol consumption include the following, among others:

- High blood pressure
- Heart disease
- Liver disease
- Memory problems
- Depression
- Anxiety

Some people are also more susceptible to problems from alcohol, meaning how alcohol affects you may be different from someone else. Some of the factors that account for variation are gender, age, family history of alcohol-related problems, ethnicity, health status, whether it was consumed slowly or quickly, and if food is eaten with the alcohol.

Plus, unfortunately, there are additional health risks associated with drinking and diabetes, even if you don't drink excessively. Alcohol can make your blood glucose more difficult to control by causing it to go higher or lower. It is especially important to follow alcohol safety guidelines if you take insulin or certain diabetes medications (such as glipizide, glyburide, glimepiride, repaglinide, or nateglinide) to decrease the risk of hypoglycemia, which can occur up to 24 hours after drinking. Symptoms of hypoglycemia—dizziness, lack of coordination, and disorientation—can be mistaken for having too much to drink, making the situation particularly dangerous.

Another downside with alcohol and diabetes that may contribute to both hyperglycemia and weight gain is how alcohol can affect your eating. When drinking, you may find it harder to not overeat. The alcohol itself adds extra calories with no nutritional value. If you don't stay on track with your eating, you may end up overindulging on extra snacks, desserts, or overly large food portions.

Potential Benefits from Alcohol

As far as heart health goes, moderate consumption of any type of alcohol can increase your HDL or "good" cholesterol, which is protective against heart disease. Light to moderate drinkers also tend to live longer than people who don't drink any alcohol, though research is ongoing on this. Another interesting find from observational studies is that women who are moderate drinkers actually have higher bone density than those who don't drink alcohol.

One particular alcoholic drink you've probably heard being touted as beneficial to your health is wine, particularly red wine. In fact, there are several compounds in red wine that may decrease the risk of heart disease. Resveratrol was thought by scientists to be the main beneficial substance in red wine, as a result of studies showing positive health benefits in mice. Because of this, resveratrol started being promoted in the media with a variety of health claims; it was "the" *antioxidant* that would put an end to heart disease, prevent cancer, and slow down the aging process! However, more recent studies have shed additional light that resveratrol on its own may not be as beneficial as early research indicated. Luckily, there are other advantageous compounds in red wine that may work best in combination with resveratrol. And for people with type 2 diabetes, light to moderate consumption of alcohol, particularly wine, has been shown to decrease risk of dying from a heart attack.

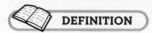 **DEFINITION**

An **antioxidant** is a substance that protects the body's cells from damage caused by oxygenation. Vitamin C and vitamin E are examples of antioxidants.

While you don't want to start drinking just because you might gain some health benefits, if you choose to continue drinking alcohol, we recommend the following guidelines:

- Only drink alcohol when your blood glucose is in good control.

- Don't drink on an empty stomach. Have food with alcohol.

- Drink water along with alcohol to stay hydrated and to slow down your alcohol intake.

- Don't skip food to make up the extra calories from alcohol.

- If you like mixed drinks, to lower the carbohydrates, choose low- or no-calorie mixers like diet tonic water, diet soda, club soda, or sparkling water. Sweet drinks can raise your blood glucose.

- When drinking alcohol, check your blood glucose more frequently. Before you drink, if you feel your blood sugar is low, and before you go to bed are good times to check. A blood glucose level of 100 to 140 mg/dL is generally safe at bedtime. Ask your medical provider if this is a good target for you.

As you're considering whether to continue drinking based on the benefits we've shared, don't forget that the bigger picture of your eating pattern and lifestyle has quite a bit of influence on your overall health. If you're a couch potato who eats mainly fast food, for example, you won't see the same benefit from alcohol as a person who has an active lifestyle and eats sensibly. So the bottom line is if you drink alcohol, drink only in moderation and continue to eat a variety of healthful foods in order to benefit.

Smoking

If you smoke, you already know it's not good for you. There are no health gains or upsides with smoking. If you've tried quitting, you know it is not easy. The main reason it is so difficult to give up smoking is the nicotine. Nicotine affects your lungs, brain, blood vessels, heart, and how you metabolize food. And according to the American Cancer Society, nicotine not only causes physical dependence, it also affects you emotionally. Because of the enjoyable feelings nicotine causes, it makes you want to smoke more. The more and the longer you smoke, the more nicotine you need to get the same pleasant feelings. The nicotine level drops as soon as a cigarette is finished, and a craving for another can start right away. Plus, uncomfortable feelings can increase if smoking is put off for a long period of time and only relieved by another cigarette.

When it comes to smoking and diabetes, smokers are 30 to 40 percent more likely to develop type 2 diabetes, according to the CDC. The risk goes up the more you smoke. If you have type 2 diabetes and smoke, high levels of nicotine make it more difficult to control your blood glucose. Because nicotine causes insulin to not work as well, higher doses of insulin are needed to manage diabetes for smokers compared to nonsmokers. Diabetes complications are also more likely due to the negative effects of smoking on the body. For people with diabetes, smoking increases the risk of amputations, heart attacks or stroke, end-stage kidney disease (dialysis), and blindness.

Benefits of Not Smoking

The risks we've mentioned can all improve if you quit. If you've smoked for a long time, you may think it's too late to get benefits from quitting smoking. That's not true. Quality of life improves after quitting at most any age. While quitting when you're younger further lengthens your life expectancy, even older adults who've smoked for years can become healthier and feel better after they quit. As an ex-smoker, you will have a lower risk of getting cold and flu viruses and be less likely to have bronchitis and pneumonia than smokers. Wait, there's more! After you quit, you'll have a lower risk of having a heart attack or stroke and a decreased risk of lung cancer and chronic lung diseases.

The time frame when you start experiencing benefits also starts sooner than you think. Some short-term benefits include the following:

- Improved sense of taste and smell

- Fresher breath

- Lack of yellow stains on your fingernails

- Fresher-smelling clothes and hair

- Increased energy and lung capacity

Making such a significant change can also make you feel better about yourself. Taking on this type of challenge and conquering it can do a lot for your self-esteem. Sounds like quitting time!

 FOR YOUR SAFETY

Smoking can affect the way your body uses certain medications. Because you can clear out some drugs more quickly than if you didn't smoke, quitting may affect the amount of medication that stays in your system. Ask your medical provider if you need a different dose of any of your medications after you quit smoking.

Smoking Withdrawal

When you try to cut back or quit smoking, the decrease in nicotine leads to withdrawal symptoms. Even if you've only smoked regularly for a few weeks, withdrawal symptoms can occur when you stop. These symptoms may include the following:

- Sore throat

- Dry mouth

- Chest tightness

- Slower heart rate

- Difficulty sleeping

- Headaches

- Fatigue

- Hunger

- Weight gain

- Constipation

Along with these physical symptoms, emotionally you may feel depressed, anxious, irritable, restless, or distracted. Withdrawal symptoms can start soon after the last cigarette and last up to several weeks. It takes about two to three days for most of the nicotine to leave the body. However, the longer you go without smoking, the more the symptoms improve.

If you want to quit successfully, you need to be prepared to deal with the physical and emotional aspects of quitting. To increase the odds of success, plan a "quit day" and tell people close to you about it to gain support. Also, ask your medical provider about tools to help you quit, such as nicotine patches or medications. You can find a number of resources to help you quit smoking in Appendix B.

Combating Weight Gain When Quitting

Has worry about weight gain stopped you from quitting smoking? If so, you'll be glad to know that you don't automatically have to pack on any pounds when you quit. Not everyone gains weight, and the amount of weight gained is usually smaller than you imagine. The reason weight gain is common after quitting is because smoking makes you less hungry and slightly increases your metabolism. Because nicotine speeds up your heart rate, you burn more calories, but not in a good way. After you stop smoking, your appetite and metabolism go back to normal. Being hungrier and having an improved sense of smell and taste may potentially contribute to overeating if you're not careful. Instead, if you slow down your eating and savor the flavors, you can enjoy your newly improved senses without going overboard. However, tackling the nicotine addiction should be your number-one priority. So when you're ready to quit, focus on quitting, not dieting. After all, drastic changes aren't needed to prevent weight gain.

DIABETES DECODED

Smoking increases metabolism by about 10 percent, or approximately 200 calories per day. To remove 100 calories from your food intake, eat only half a bagel, choose nonfat milk instead of whole milk, substitute ham in place of bacon or sausage at breakfast, or leave the pepperoni off your pizza. To burn off 100 more calories (for a 150-pound person), go bowling for 30 minutes, dance for 20 minutes, briskly walk for 20 minutes, or swim for 15 minutes. Together, these small changes can make a big difference!

One of the best things you can do to avoid weight gain and help you quit smoking is to increase your physical activity. Most people can add walking somewhere into their day—even 10 minutes at a time can help. This will not only help you burn more calories, but it will also help fight the depression and anxiety that can come with quitting (see Chapter 7 for more ideas to increase physical activity).

The following are some tips to help you stay on track with your eating plan while quitting smoking:

- Drink water throughout the day. This helps you feel full and can decrease the urge to smoke.

- Eat more vegetables. When you feel like grabbing a cigarette, grab a carrot, celery stick, sliced green pepper, or cherry tomato instead.

- Nibble on some low-calorie, low-carbohydrate choices for sweet cravings. Choose sugar-free breath mints, gum, popsicles, or lollipops. Just don't overdo it with the sugar-free treats as they may cause discomfort due to gas and bloating.

- Try hobbies or activities that make it difficult for you to eat (or smoke!). Painting your nails, knitting, playing a musical instrument, writing a letter, petting your dog, or working on model cars are all things that keep your hands busy.

The most important thing is to not let a fear of weight gain keep you from quitting. If you end up gaining a few pounds, you can deal with that later as a nonsmoker!

Taking Supplements

To say that *dietary supplements* are popular in the United States is quite an understatement. Approximately half of American adults take supplements primarily to improve or maintain their health. In 2002, it was reported that people with diabetes are 1.6 times more likely to use supplements than people without diabetes.

Are there supplements that really help control diabetes? Well, it turns out there are more claims about these natural remedies than actual evidence. The Food and Drug Administration (FDA) oversees dietary supplement products using a different set of rules than for either conventional drugs or food ingredients. Unlike medications, manufacturers of dietary supplements don't have to prove to the FDA the products are safe and effective before selling them; instead, the businesses are responsible for safety and accurate labeling of their own products. If an issue about safety or false labeling is reported after the product is on the market, only then is the FDA responsible for taking action. What this means is that claims regarding supplements can be wide ranging and not as easy to verify as with medications. That's why medical professionals may not be as quick to recommend dietary supplements as people with diabetes are to try them.

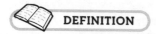 **DEFINITION**

> **Dietary supplements** are products in pill, liquid, or powder form people take by mouth to increase the nutritional value of their usual diet. Dietary ingredients included in supplements are vitamins, minerals, or herbs, among others.

To help you become more supplement savvy, we're going to talk about the most common supplements used by people with diabetes and whether they're worth trying. While some supplements may have looked favorable to help manage diabetes in early research but have not held up well under the spotlight, others are rising to the top with promising potential. Talk with your medical provider before starting a supplement to make sure it's safe for you.

Vitamin D

With all the media coverage about vitamin D over the past few years, you have probably heard or read something about this unique vitamin. Unlike other vitamins that have to be consumed, vitamin D is different because it is made by your body with help from the sun. That's why vitamin D is referred to as the "sunshine" vitamin. To make enough vitamin D, your skin (not just your face and arms) needs to be exposed to the sun for about 10 to 15 minutes a day. Due to skin cancer risk, many people use sunscreen, which decreases vitamin D production. Some guidelines recommend waiting 10 minutes before putting on sunscreen to counteract this effect.

Those who live in less sunny places with colder weather generally have lower levels of vitamin D in their blood due to less sun exposure.

Not many foods contain vitamin D. Fatty fish like salmon, mackerel, and tuna are good sources, with smaller amounts available in beef liver, sardines, and egg yolks. And Grandma's often-recommended health remedy, cod-liver oil, is an excellent source of vitamin D. (But you would need way more than "a spoonful of sugar" to make it taste good!) Some foods have vitamin D added; in those cases, you'll see "vitamin D fortified" on the label. Milk, soy milk, orange juice, yogurt, cheese, margarine, and breakfast cereals are commonly fortified with vitamin D. Unless you regularly include these foods in your eating plan, it can be difficult to get enough vitamin D to keep the vitamin D levels in your blood high enough.

Vitamin D is important for your health because it helps you use calcium to strengthen your bones and prevent osteoporosis. It also plays a role in heart health by regulating the amount of calcium in your blood. Your immune system even depends on vitamin D to do its job, warding off potential infections and viruses.

 FOR YOUR SAFETY

Excessive amounts of vitamin D can be toxic. If you have too much vitamin D in your blood, it can cause nausea, confusion, constipation, kidney stones, and disturbances in your heart rhythm. The recommended maximum upper limit for adults is 4,000 IU per day, with 1,000 to 2,000 IU per day from supplements.

When it comes to diabetes in particular, a number of studies have indicated there is a connection between low levels of vitamin D and type 2 diabetes. Vitamin D has been linked to the development of type 2 diabetes, with low blood levels of vitamin D increasing the risk. Having the right amount of vitamin D may also be important in blood glucose control once you have type 2 diabetes. (More research about type 2 diabetes and vitamin D is underway.)

The good news is that vitamin D supplements are considered safe and effective. They come in two forms: D_2 and D_3. The D_3 type is the most commonly available and is generally preferred. As for dosage, there has been some controversy in the medical field about just how much vitamin D to recommend. Currently, the Institute of Medicine (IOM) recommends 600 international units (IU) daily for adults through age 70 and 800 IU ages 71 and above.

Talk with your medical provider about checking your blood to see if you are one of the many with low vitamin D levels. If supplements are recommended, your medical provider should tell you about the best dose and what type is right for you. You may just get the boost you need for better blood glucose management with vitamin D.

CoQ10

CoQ10, also known as coenzyme Q10, is an antioxidant present in your body cells that helps make energy and uses oxygen to prevent damage to the cells. Good food sources of CoQ10 include fatty fish like salmon and tuna, liver, and whole grains.

As a supplement, this antioxidant has been promoted to help with heart disease, high blood pressure, fertility, gum disease, Parkinson's disease, migraines, and diabetes, among other conditions. However, the results of studies on CoQ10 for diabetes control are mixed. While several controlled trials of CoQ10 in people with type 1 and type 2 diabetes did not show improvements in blood glucose or a decrease in insulin dosing, another controlled trial found improved blood glucose control over time, as well as better blood pressure in participants with type 2 diabetes.

CoQ10 supplements are generally thought to be safe, though there may be some side effects, which include the following:

- Nausea
- Diarrhea
- Stomach upset
- Vomiting
- Heartburn

When used as a supplement, doses range from 30 to 200 mg per day. Some medications may interact with CoQ10. For example, CoQ10 may decrease how well blood-thinning drugs like warfarin (Coumadin) and clpidigrel (Plavix) work. Plus, some medications, such as statin drugs for cholesterol, lower the amount of CoQ10 in your body. If you take these medications, it is especially important that you talk with your medical provider about whether taking CoQ10 is safe and effective for you.

Magnesium

Magnesium is necessary for numerous functions in your body. Just some of the functions that magnesium supports are nerve and muscle function, a healthy immune system, a regular heart rate, strong bones, and blood glucose control. People who eat more magnesium are less likely to develop type 2 diabetes, and it continues to play a key role in regulating blood glucose when you have diabetes.

Good food sources of magnesium include whole grains, nuts, pumpkin seeds, leafy green vegetables, potatoes, avocados, and dried beans (such as kidney and black beans). If you regularly include these food sources and take a multivitamin, you may be getting all the magnesium you need.

However, approximately one out of four people with diabetes may have low magnesium levels. When your blood glucose is high, your kidneys put out more urine, and magnesium is lost along with the urine. Diuretics, also called *water pills,* can increase magnesium loss, too. Low blood levels of magnesium in turn can worsen insulin resistance and decrease insulin secreted by the pancreas, making blood glucose even more difficult to control. Due to this magnesium loss, supplements may be recommended.

 DIABETES DECODED

> The letters *USP* on the label of a dietary supplement indicate the product has been independently tested to ensure quality and accuracy and meets FDA standards. This is a voluntary process for manufacturers that ensures the product contains what it says it does on the label, dissolves to become available for digestion, and is the strength listed. If not independently tested, you're taking the manufacturer's word that the label is accurate.

Ask your medical provider if you should have your magnesium levels checked. If your blood levels of magnesium are low, you may benefit from correcting that through magnesium supplements. The recommended daily intake for men is 400 mg a day for ages 19 to 30 and 420 mg after age 30. For women, 310 mg is recommended for ages 19 to 30 and 320 mg after age 30.

Talk with your medical provider before you supplement magnesium on your own. In higher doses, magnesium may cause diarrhea. If you have kidney disease, the amount of magnesium in your blood may go up too high; in that case, you wouldn't want to take extra. Plus too much magnesium can affect your heart rhythm and cause low blood pressure.

Alpha-Lipoic Acid

Alpha-lipoic acid, also known as lipoic acid, is an antioxidant found inside the cells in your body that helps your cells use glucose for energy. It also helps regenerate other antioxidants like vitamin C and vitamin E to ward off cell damage. It is also found in foods, with sources including red meat, liver and other organ meats, broccoli, spinach, and brewer's yeast.

Most healthy people make enough alpha-lipoic acid and don't need to supplement it. Still, study results have suggested that alpha-lipoic acid supplements may lower blood glucose by increasing insulin sensitivity. If caught early enough, before too much nerve damage is done, alpha-lipoic acid may also be helpful in decreasing symptoms of diabetic neuropathy, such as tingling, numbness, pain, or burning sensation in the feet and legs. While the results are promising, additional studies are needed to confirm these benefits.

Alpha-lipoic acid supplements may add to the effect of diabetes medications to lower blood glucose, so you'll need to test your blood glucose more frequently to prevent hypoglycemia if you start taking it. The dose for alpha-lipoic acid has not been set because there's no proven treatment using this supplement. Research studies have been conducted using daily doses ranging from 600 to 1,200 mg. While some suggest there is evidence that a three-week oral daily dose of 600 mg is effective for the treatment of diabetic neuropathy symptoms, many of the studies on alpha-lipoic acid are with intravenous (IV) treatment rather than pills. Additional studies need to be conducted to see if the same effects are seen with oral supplements as with IV therapy. Caution should be used with high doses, as heart rhythm problems could occur. The higher the dose, the more likely you could have side effects.

If your medical provider recommends using an alpha-lipoic acid supplement, the dose of your diabetes medication may need to be adjusted to prevent hypoglycemia. Alpha-lipoic acid also may lower levels of thyroid hormone. If you're taking thyroid medication such as levothyroxine, your medical provider may need to monitor your thyroid function more closely. Other potential side effects of taking alpha-lipoic acid are skin rash and upset stomach.

Cinnamon

What is better to put on your oatmeal in the morning than a sprinkle of cinnamon? Cinnamon adds a natural sweetness to foods and can help to reduce the amount of sugar you need when baking. While there are different types of cinnamon, cassia cinnamon is commonly found on grocery store shelves and is the type that's been studied for its blood glucose–lowering effects.

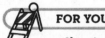 **FOR YOUR SAFETY**

If you're currently taking supplements, make sure to share that information with both your medical provider and the pharmacy where you fill your prescriptions. They can help identify potential reactions between your prescription medications and supplements before it's too late.

As a supplement, cinnamon has mixed results. A number of clinical studies have looked at the effect of cinnamon on blood glucose control in people with type 2 diabetes. Some of the studies showed promising results, while others didn't show any benefit. So the evidence is not conclusive. Interestingly, in a study showing positive results, the smallest amount of cinnamon used—1 g or approximately $1/2$ teaspoon of cinnamon daily—showed the best blood glucose–lowering results. Other studies have used varying amounts of cinnamon.

When large doses are taken over a longer time period, cassia cinnamon may not be safe. A substance called *coumarin*, which is present in cassia cinnamon, has been linked to liver damage in some people. If you have liver disease, you should avoid taking cassia cinnamon. If you and your medical provider decide you should try taking a cinnamon supplement to improve blood glucose control, start with the lowest dose shown to be effective—1 g (given as 500 mg twice daily)—and closely monitor your blood glucose.

Zinc

You might not have heard much about zinc, except possibly that it's in products designed to fight off colds and the flu. Those products contain zinc because it plays a key role in strengthening the immune system. Zinc also helps with growth and development, wound healing, your sense of taste and smell, and other body functions. Zinc is necessary for insulin production in the pancreas and is needed for the process to break down carbohydrates into glucose for energy. Zinc is also an essential mineral you need to get from food. Food sources of zinc include oysters, seafood, meats, chicken and turkey, dairy products, legumes, nuts, and whole grains.

Low blood levels of zinc have been associated with an increased risk of type 2 diabetes. Symptoms of zinc deficiency include low insulin levels, poor appetite, irritability, hair loss, rough and dry skin, slow wound healing, poor sense of taste and smell, diarrhea, and nausea.

Increased zinc intake from food sources may decrease type 2 diabetes risk. However, studies examining the role of zinc supplements on blood glucose control have shown mixed results—some saw improvement, while others did not.

Not much zinc is needed to meet requirements; adult men need 11 mg daily, and adult women need 8 mg per day. So choosing foods high in zinc and taking a multivitamin/mineral supplement should get you more than enough. While zinc supplements up to 40 mg per day are considered safe, too much zinc may affect copper levels in your body. High doses of zinc may also cause stomach pain, coughing, fatigue, and other issues. Either high doses of zinc, or long-term use at lower doses, may increase the risk of prostate cancer in men. Zinc supplements can also decrease the effectiveness of some antibiotics. Talk to your medical provider if you're thinking about using a zinc supplement.

FOR YOUR SAFETY

Using a supplement doesn't take the place of eating a variety fruits and vegetables, whole grains, low-fat or nonfat dairy products, and lean protein. What you eat and how active you are still matter. No diabetes supplement or medication can replace you as a diabetes manager.

Chromium

Chromium is an essential mineral that's needed only in small amounts in the body. Chromium seems to enhance the action of insulin and is directly involved in the breakdown of carbohydrates, protein, and fat for energy. Chromium can be found in small amounts in many foods, including broccoli, potatoes, whole-grain breads, brewer's yeast, grape juice, and beef, among others. You also get chromium from tap water and cooking in stainless-steel pots.

Low chromium intake has been linked with insulin resistance, elevated triglycerides and cholesterol, and increased risk of diabetes and heart disease. Exactly how chromium works and the amounts needed for optimum health status aren't well defined. However, the recommended daily intake of chromium for nonpregnant adults ranges from 20 to 35 micrograms (mcg), depending on gender and age. Increased chromium—up to 45 mcg—is needed during pregnancy and while breastfeeding.

Chromium, in the form of the supplement chromium picolinate, has been widely studied as a potential treatment for diabetes. Studies using chromium for type 2 diabetes included doses from 200 to 1,000 mcg. Early studies showed promise as to its effectiveness in blood glucose control. More recent studies show that maybe only certain people respond to chromium supplements, perhaps those that are deficient. However, chromium deficiency is difficult to detect because amounts in the blood, urine, and hair don't necessarily indicate body stores of this trace mineral. Improvement in blood glucose control in people with type 2 diabetes remains inconclusive.

Chromium supplements are typically considered safe for most adults in daily doses up to 1,000 mcg up to six months. However, longer-term use of chromium may increase the risk of side effects. While side effects from chromium supplements are rare, excessive chromium supplementation may cause stomach problems; hypoglycemia; liver, kidney, or nerve damage; and irregular heart rhythm. Close blood glucose monitoring is recommended when using chromium supplements along with diabetes medication or insulin.

Tips for Supplement Use

Now that you know some of the risks and potential benefits of common diabetes related supplements, there are a few extra things to get the best benefit from a supplement you've selected to try.

Review your decision with your medical provider to determine that the supplement is safe to take, based on your personal health history and medications. If you've been given the green light, make sure you understand both the benefits and the risks of taking that particular supplement.

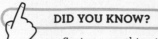 **DID YOU KNOW?**

Saying something is natural doesn't mean it's safe. There are many things that are both natural and harmful at the same time—for example, poisonous mushrooms.

Give the supplement time to work. For example, if you're taking a supplement to improve blood glucose control, give it about two to three months. If your next A1C test doesn't show improvement, you may need to try something else.

Ask your medical provider if lab tests to check your kidney and liver functions are recommended while taking a supplement. Many medications and supplements affect the kidneys and liver because of how they are cleared out of the body.

Stick with the recommended dose of the supplement. More is not better. Mega doses are more likely to cause unwanted side effects or be harmful.

Find out whether it's necessary to interrupt your supplement schedule. For example, some supplements may need to be stopped temporarily prior to surgery because they increase the risk of bleeding or affect how you respond to anesthesia.

Choose supplements that are made by a trusted manufacturer. Brand-name and store-brand supplements are both fine, as long as it is a brand or store that is trustworthy. Major brands are more likely to adhere to standards of good manufacturing practices and be truthful in promoting a product.

The Least You Need to Know

- Most people with diabetes can drink moderate amounts of alcohol. However, excessive alcohol intake can have serious health risks and negatively affect blood glucose control.

- When you have diabetes, smoking is even more harmful than if you don't have diabetes. Therefore, quitting is the only option for protecting your health.

- Talk with your medical provider before starting a supplement and make sure you understand the potential side effects and benefits of it.

The Importance of Sleeping and Coping with Stress

If you check your blood glucose and the result is higher than usual, probably the first two things you think about are what you ate and if you took your medication as planned. However, you may not think about how you slept the night before or how stressed you are. You'd be surprised at the impact that sleep and stress can also have on your blood glucose.

Poor sleep and stress can contribute to high blood glucose individually and together, with lack of sleep feeding stress and vice versa. So in this chapter, we discuss how getting better sleep and taking time to relax can improve your overall health and diabetes management.

In This Chapter

- How sleep affects your blood glucose

- Improving your chances for a restful sleep

- The effects of stress on your body

- Relaxation and stress management techniques

Why Sleep Is Important

When you were a child, you were probably reminded on a regular basis about the importance of rest and sleep with phrases like "get a good night's sleep," "night night, sleep tight," and "sleep well." As an adult, sleep is still very important, but if you're like a lot of people, you probably don't get enough. The CDC estimates that up to 70 million adults in the United States have sleep or wakefulness disorders. Lack of sleep has been linked to risks of becoming obese and getting type 2 diabetes. Fatigue may contribute to overeating due to the belief that eating will boost energy. Plus, the foods selected tend to be less nutritious options, providing empty calories and leading to weight gain. Some studies have also shown that lack of sleep leads to insulin resistance, which can turn into type 2 diabetes over time, if not treated. People who have diabetes may not sleep as much, or as well, as people without diabetes. High blood glucose can lead to frequent urination which can cause multiple trips to the bathroom in the middle of the night. Obesity and type 2 diabetes are also risk factors for sleep apnea, which causes poor sleep quality (more on that later in this chapter). As you age, sleep quality also declines.

So how much sleep should you get? It's all about finding the right balance for yourself; you want a sleep that's both restful and long enough without being too long. Let's take a look at what you need to get a good night's sleep.

Getting Enough Sleep

While not everyone needs the same amount of sleep, seven to nine hours seems to be about the right amount for the majority of adults. If you aren't getting that amount of sleep, there are some things you can do to help yourself catch more shut-eye. The most important way to better control your sleep schedule is by getting to bed at a regular time. You have a built-in sleep-wake cycle that tells your body when to get up and when to go to bed, making it hard for your body to switch gears when you change up your sleep schedule. This could be due to sleeping in late on the weekends and getting up early on the weekdays, working varying shifts, or traveling across time zones. By going to bed and getting up close to the same time each day, you help yourself stay on track with your sleep.

Beyond a proper sleep schedule, here are some tips for getting enough sleep:

- **Don't participate in physical activity too close to your bedtime.** While staying active is a plus for diabetes management, try to finish your exercise at least two to three hours before bed. That way, you're not energized and awake when you go to bed.

- **Kick the afternoon caffeine.** It may take up to eight hours for caffeine to get out of your system, so any afternoon coffee, cola, or tea may still be having an effect when you go to bed.

- **Don't eat too much before bed.** A small snack is fine, but eating a large meal may cause heartburn and discomfort that could keep you awake.

- **Don't nap too late or too long.** While quick naps can help you feel rested and more focused, make sure you don't nap after 3 P.M. and keep them to 30 minutes or less; otherwise, you may negatively affect your sleep at night.

- **Make your room conducive to sleep.** Because light makes your body think it's time to get up, your room should be dark when you're sleeping. Your room should also be comfortable in terms of noise and temperature—not uncomfortably hot, cold, or noisy.

- **Create a bedtime routine.** Make a plan to allow some time to unwind at the end of the day. Relax before bed by reading or listening to music (just not while in bed!).

 DIABETES DECODED

Checking emails, browsing the internet, watching television, playing video games, texting, and other "screen" time before you go to bed can cause you to stay up later than you planned. Plus, the light exposure from the screen (computer, cell phones, tablet devices, and so on) can decrease the hormone melatonin, which tells your brain when it's time to sleep. Sleep experts recommend making your bedroom a technology-free zone. If you can't get away from it entirely, shut off the technology at least 15 minutes before you go to bed—an hour is better.

How Well Do You Sleep?

Sleep isn't just about quantity, though; it's also about quality. How do you know if you're having quality sleep? The following lists some common signs of lack of sleep quality:

- It takes you over 30 minutes to fall asleep at bedtime.

- You wake up in the night and can't get back to sleep.

- You wake up earlier than you want to.

- You fall asleep during the day at unplanned times. (This is especially dangerous if you've fallen asleep while driving.)

- You rely on caffeinated beverages to stay awake during the day.

There are a number of factors, both internal and external, which affect how well you sleep. Various medical conditions—such as chronic pain and anxiety—can disrupt your slumber. If you're not sleeping well at night due to uncontrolled pain or anxiety, talk with your medical provider about potential treatment options. There are other nonpharmaceutical options for both pain control and anxiety, so don't feel the only solution is to take another pill.

Medications may also be the cause of restless nights. If you're taking a number of prescription medications and sleeping has become a problem, ask your medical provider or pharmacist if any of your prescriptions might be keeping you awake at night. Potential solutions include using a different drug with fewer side effects, or you may be able to take your medication earlier in the day to avoid wakefulness.

Certain behaviors can also lead to poor sleep. For instance, alcohol and quality sleep don't mix. If you have more than one or two drinks, you may fall asleep but stay in the lighter stages of sleep, meaning you're not getting the deep sleep you need. Drinking can also cause nighttime hypoglycemia or contribute to high fasting blood sugar. Waking up in the middle of the night is also a problem after drinking alcohol. Not only do you get up to go to the bathroom more, but once the effects of the alcohol wear off, you tend to wake up. If you really want a good night's sleep, forgo the alcohol. Smoking is also bad for sleep. Nicotine is a stimulant, which can make it difficult for you to fall asleep. Like alcohol, smoking can also cause you to spend more time in light sleep than nonsmokers, affecting the quality of your sleep. Plus, nicotine withdrawal symptoms can happen overnight or just prior to waking, which if you recall can lead to discomfort and make you less likely to stay asleep. If sleep is important to you, this may be the reason for you to choose to quit smoking.

If you have any of the signs occur frequently, try all the tips for getting a better night's sleep. If you're still having reoccurring signs of sleep deprivation, you may need to talk with your medical provider about it.

Obstructive Sleep Apnea

Have you gone through all of the previous recommendations and still been unable to get a good night's rest? If you have type 2 diabetes and you're having difficulty sleeping, *obstructive sleep apnea (OSA)* is a prime suspect. A number of studies have shown a strong connection between type 2 diabetes and OSA. Most common in middle-aged, overweight men, people with OSA have double the risk of developing type 2 diabetes than those without OSA, and approximately half of men who already have diabetes also have OSA. Several recent studies have indicated that as OSA becomes more severe, insulin sensitivity decreases, causing insulin resistance. OSA causes lack of oxygen, increased levels of circulating stress hormones, and inflammation, which are triggers for insulin resistance.

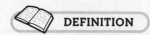 **DEFINITION**

Obstructive sleep apnea (OSA) is a chronic condition that causes a temporary stoppage in breathing during sleep. Symptoms can include loud snoring with pauses and loud snorting or choking sounds when breathing starts again.

With OSA, the muscles at the base of your tongue and the back of your throat relax and block off the airway, temporarily stopping breathing. Snoring indicates that air is being forced through a partial blockage, while a stoppage in snoring usually indicates a complete blockage of the airway. This can happen repeatedly throughout the night, jolting you awake (or at least partially awake). You then end up staying in light sleep without beneficial deep, restorative sleep. When you wake up, you tend to still feel tired and sleepy, a feeling that carries throughout the day. This form of sleep deprivation may contribute to memory changes, depression, and irritability. Physically, OSA decreases oxygen in your blood, increases your blood pressure, and puts stress on your heart.

Not sure you have OSA or other sleep problems that should be checked out? The following are some signs that may mean you're having more than just a bit of trouble sleeping:

- When you first wake up, you feel like you just can't move.

- Your sleeping partner tells you that you make jerking movements with your legs or arms during sleep.

- You have vivid dreams when you're falling asleep or even dozing.

- Your sleeping partner reports that you snore loudly, make choking noises, or snort in your sleep, or notices that you stop breathing for short periods.

- Even after sleeping seven or eight hours, you don't feel well rested.

The good thing is that OSA and other sleep disorders can be treated, so don't avoid the discussion just because you think it can't be helped. If you have any of the preceding signs of OSA (or suspect you have some other sleep disorder), schedule an appointment with your medical provider and share that you have difficulty sleeping. Generally, your provider will order a sleep study to determine if you have OSA or another sleep disorder and then, based on the results, together with your provider, you can determine the best treatment option for you.

Fighting Stress

Stress; where would you be without it? While picturing a life without stress sounds wonderful, having no stress at all would actually be quite boring. And stress doesn't just happen with the bad stuff—it happens with the good things, too. While having to take a test, getting stuck in traffic, and getting sick or injured are probably the kinds of stressors you would just as soon do without, getting married, having a baby, and buying a new house are sources of positive stress.

Having to live with stress, both positive and negative, is something everyone does. What varies is how people cope with stress, or how they manage it. Some coping techniques don't help actually manage the stress—or improve blood glucose control. For example, reaching for a cigarette, alcohol, or half-gallon of ice cream (or candy bars, chips, donuts, and so on) isn't the most effective coping technique, but it tends to be what people do. So learning effective strategies to better manage your stress not only helps you deal with day-to-day challenges, it also helps with your overall health and diabetes control.

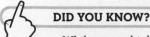

DID YOU KNOW?

While many think of stress as simply emotional, stress can be physical, too. Examples of physical stress include being sick with the flu or having surgery.

Why Stress Affects Blood Sugar

When it comes to stress, your body doesn't know the difference between a real threat or an imagined one. Therefore, your body prepares you to face the threat by releasing "stress hormones" called *epinephrine* and *cortisol*. These hormones make your heart beat faster, increase your blood pressure, make you breathe more quickly, and raise your blood glucose so you have enough energy to either meet the danger head on or get away from it (also known as "fight or flight"). When you don't have diabetes, your body is able to respond by lowering your blood glucose when it's not really needed. But with diabetes, your body doesn't compensate as well to get your blood glucose back down; instead, your blood glucose stays elevated, even when the perceived threat is over.

So does that mean all stress is bad? No; short bursts of stress are actually helpful. For instance, the stress of a deadline may help you get your work done sooner and help you stay focused on your task. Stress can also help you avoid danger like when you pull your hand away from a hot stove. However, it's important for you to understand what stress feels like to you and to note physical and emotional symptoms. If you're in tune to how stress affects you, you can take steps to manage it before it gets out of control. Taking note of your stress level when you test your blood glucose will help you discover what stressors cause elevations.

Even when you're monitoring your stress levels, chronic stress can still sneak up on you, and you don't always realize the negative effects it's having on you until you become overwhelmed. Stress may trigger high blood glucose and high blood pressure, increase the risk of heart attack and stroke, and suppress your immune system. Emotionally, you may have increased anxiety and depression. But it's hard to say how much stress is too much. Everyone's stress limit is different. Some people will feel completely overloaded with a situation that others might actually seek out. However, if you're developing some of the following symptoms, it's a signal that your stress level is out of control and you need to take action to regain control. Symptoms of uncontrolled stress include the following:

- Worried and anxious thoughts

- Changes in appetite (eating too much or not enough)

- Significant weight loss or gain

- Teeth grinding

- Trouble with memory and concentration, and difficulty completing tasks

- Sleeping too much or not enough

- Irritability, anger, and frustration

- Stomach problems (such as nausea, constipation, and diarrhea)

- Headaches

- Trembling and shakiness

- Profuse sweating

- Depression

If you're experiencing symptoms of uncontrolled stress, talk with your medical provider. Your medical provider can make referrals to the appropriate specialist if needed.

DIABETES DECODED

Depression is common with diabetes and directly linked to type 2 diabetes. If you're unsure whether you're depressed, you can use these two questions as a screening tool to check for depression risk:

1. During the past month, have you often been bothered by feeling down, depressed, or hopeless?

2. During the past month, have you found you have little interest or pleasure in doing things?

If you answered "yes" to either of these questions, make an appointment with your medical provider to get further assessment for depression. Depression can worsen diabetes control and high blood glucose can contribute to depression, leading to a vicious cycle. Therefore, it's important to seek help to break this cycle.

The Four "A"s of Stress Management

In any given stressful situation, there are basically four things you can do. They are the four "A"s of stress management: avoid, alter, accept, or adapt. You may use any or all of these options successfully, depending on the scenario, in order to manage your stress level and in turn manage your health. Let's take a look at each option and some examples of how they work.

Avoid: There are actually a number of stressors you can just choose to avoid so you don't have to deal with them. The following are different ways you can avoid a stressful situation:

- If you really can't take on another activity, it is okay to say no. For example, if you can't coach your son's Little League team, you can be a good cheerleader for him at the games. One of the best lines you can learn to use is "No, thank you; I'm overcommitted."

- If busy traffic on your commute really annoys you, find an alternate route or leave earlier for work.

- If the ads on television bother you, shut the TV off and read a book. Or if you're not ready to give up your show because of ads just yet, you can mute the sound on the ads and walk around your living room until your show is back on.

Alter: Of course, not all stress can be avoided. If possible, you can change your situation so it works for you. The following illustrate how a stressful situation can be altered:

- Prioritize and get just the important things done today. You don't have to complete everything on your list every day. For instance, you can choose not to organize your desk today; it can wait until tomorrow.

- Practice good communication skills. Sometimes avoiding having a conversation just makes it blow way out of proportion. Using the describe, explain, specify, and consequence technique (see Chapter 5) can help you avoid conflict while still getting your point across.

- Find the positive people at work, where you volunteer, or in social situations and hang out with them. Being around people with optimistic outlooks can help you change your viewpoint for the better, too.

Accept: Sometimes you just have to accept the way things are. Remember, accepting is not the same thing as giving up; it's simply acknowledging and dealing with the stressor at hand. The following are some ways you can manage stress through acceptance:

- Choose to let go of the negative feelings. Remember, no one can make you feel anything. You choose how you feel; there's always a choice. Being caught up in the stress just makes it harder to see that.

- Talk about it. It is okay to vent your frustrations; it just has to be at the right time with the right person. Phone a friend to talk it out, or ask your walking buddy to walk it out with you.

- Ask yourself if you can change your situation that's causing you stress. If the answer is no, it can help you move on. You can't fix everything, and it's okay to give yourself permission not to.

Adapt: An attitude adjustment can be just the thing to help you adapt to stressful situations. If you think you can't, you can't. If you think you can, who's going to stop you? The following examples show how you can adapt:

- Stop the negative thoughts. Choose positive affirmation statements to say to yourself when the negative creeps in. If you hear things like "I'm such a failure," turn it around as "I learned from this," "I'm okay," or "I'm on track."

- Remember, you don't have to be perfect. You probably don't ask anyone else to be; why would you ask that of yourself? If something doesn't go exactly as planned, will anyone else really notice?

- Make a list of all the things you're grateful for—things that make you happy. You can then pull out your list and read it when you're feeling down.

 DID YOU KNOW?

One of the best things you can do to help put your stressful situation into perspective is to look outside the situation and ask yourself "Will this matter in a year or two from now?" The answer is usually "no." If it is "no," you can put it behind you more quickly.

Guided Imagery and Visualization

Guided imagery uses descriptions to direct your thoughts to create a visual image and experience that helps achieve a peaceful, focused, and relaxed state. In essence, guided imagery helps you learn the skill of creating a mental image. Usually, you listen to a recording of a script that walks you through some relaxation exercises like deep breathing and muscle relaxation. This technique has been used to help manage stress, decrease pain, promote sleep, support weight management, and even help control diabetes.

When listening to guided imagery to help you become more relaxed, you will hear a description and be asked to picture yourself in a comfortable, inviting setting, such as sitting by a cool lake or near a sandy beach. When you hear the description, try to also think of the sounds and smells you would experience in that setting. Once you're able to visualize the scene and experience the scenario, your body responds as if you are actually in that place; you feel more relaxed and comfortable. It may also help you release negative, unwanted feelings and replace them with more positive, calm ones as you're guided through the process.

A good resource for guided imagery CDs and downloadable recordings is Health Journeys (healthjourneys.com). If you're not so sure that guided imagery is right for you, you can also listen to sample recordings available on the website to see what you think.

Other Relaxation Exercises for Stress Relief

There are many relaxation exercises or techniques that can help you manage your stress. Relaxation exercises typically work by helping you increase your awareness of your body. With practice, this awareness will help you pinpoint the physical sensations of stress, like muscle tension. This will allow you to notice your stress symptoms sooner and to stop the stress before it gets out of hand. There isn't one best technique, so try out a few of the following, and then practice the ones you like best.

DID YOU KNOW?

Laughter really may be the best medicine. There is growing evidence that laughter isn't just about your sense of humor; it provides many physical benefits, too. It helps lower your blood pressure, decreases your pain, improves your mood, and strengthens your immune system. This makes laughter ideal for coping with stressful situations. So look for humor in a situation and practice smiling. Let's get you started with a joke: Why did the student eat his homework? Because the teacher told him it was a piece of cake!

Mindfulness meditation: This is an activity that focuses on awareness of breathing. To start, you sit on a cushion on the floor and, if possible, with your legs crossed and your back straight. If you can't sit on the floor, you can use a chair; the main thing is keeping good posture with your back straight. You then focus on or "follow" your breathing in and out. If your thoughts wander away from concentrating on your breathing, just get back to it once you notice. For this exercise to be most effective, you need to find a place without distractions. Once you have a quiet place for this, you may want to just practice for 5 or 10 minutes to begin with. You can gradually increase the amount of time spent focusing on your breathing with practice.

Progressive muscle relaxation: With this technique, you focus on slowly tensing and then relaxing each muscle group. This allows you to become more aware of the difference between muscle tension and relaxation. You can start with your toes and gradually move up to your head, tensing and relaxing each muscle on the way. Or you can do the opposite and start with your head and work your way down.

Want a quick muscle relaxation exercise that's easy to do? When you feel yourself tensing up at work or when you're stuck in your car at an endless red light, try this "in-the-moment" relaxation exercise:

1. Sit up straight and tall.

2. Focus on breathing in through your nose and out through your mouth slowly. Say the word *breathe* or *one* each time you slowly breathe out.

3. Think positive thoughts, smile, and choose to let go of the stress.

Yoga: You can find different types of yoga classes for different skill levels at many locations. If you're just starting out, look for hatha yoga, a general term that is usually applied to the more traditional type of yoga. Often, a local YMCA or parks and recreation department offers yoga classes if you're not sure where to find them. You don't have to already be flexible to start yoga; you'll improve your flexibility and strength with practice. However, make sure if you're just starting out to find out how to modify the moves for your fitness and flexibility level. If you're not ready to join a yoga class yet, there are numerous yoga videos you can use in your own home.

Tai-chi: Based on Chinese martial arts, this is a low-impact exercise with a series of slow, focused movements. It can be adapted for beginners and is a great activity for fit healthy people, less fit older adults, and even people recovering from surgery. This mind-body activity is proving to have multiple health benefits, including better balance and improved muscle strength and function in older adults. Most communities have tai-chi classes available through the parks and recreation department, local health clubs, or the YMCA.

No matter which of these relaxation exercises you decide to use, if any, just keep practicing and you'll get better at them. To gain the most benefit, practice the relaxation exercises in tandem with the other positive coping methods discussed in this chapter. Remember, everyone lives with stress. However, if you manage it well, it doesn't create the same problems as uncontrolled stress.

 DIABETES DECODED

If you don't feel like yoga or tai-chi are for you, almost any physical activity is helpful for stress management and blood glucose control. In the end, being more active is always a good choice!

The Least You Need to Know

- Lack of sleep has been linked to risks of becoming obese and developing type 2 diabetes.
- Having a defined sleep schedule and not eating and drinking before bed are a couple ways you can ensure a good night's sleep.
- Stress can lead to your blood glucose becoming and staying elevated when you have diabetes.
- Use the four As (avoid, alter, accept, and adapt) in conjunction with relaxation exercises to better manage your stress level.

Diabetes Medications

While some people with type 2 diabetes manage their blood glucose with meal planning and physical activity alone, many also need to take diabetes medications to achieve blood glucose targets. While insulin is always needed for people with type 1 diabetes, it is regularly used for people with type 2 as well. Insulin can be used alone or in combination with other diabetes medications.

This chapter reviews current types of insulin and diabetes medications to treat diabetes, including how they work, potential side effects, and what's good and not so good about the various drugs. We also take a sneak peek into the future with what's "in the pipeline" for new treatment options. If you've heard about insulin pumps and are curious to find out more about them, that's covered here, too.

In This Chapter

- Pills and other noninsulin diabetes medications
- Medication safety tips and side effects
- Insulin types and various ways to take it
- Insulin pumps

Diabetes Pills

As more is learned about type 2 diabetes, new drugs are in development and medication options continue to expand. Because most people don't want to take a shot when a pill might work, several pills are generally tried before starting insulin (though this is not always possible). But with so many different drugs working in different ways, it can all become quite confusing. If you start reading package inserts or look up prescription drugs on the internet, you may think you should never take any medications ever again. The list of side effects can be daunting. It can also be scary and intimidating to try to read through all that information.

Therefore, in this section, we break down the discussion based on drug types, or *drug class*, to help you gain an understanding of the benefits and risks of each. To help fill in the blanks, we also recommend asking your medical provider or your pharmacist what to expect when taking the prescribed medication. Ask for clarification between anticipated side effects and those that should alert you to a more serious problem.

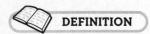

DEFINITION

> A **drug class** is a group of medications with comparable chemical structure that work in a similar way. Typically, they are used to treat the same health issue.

All medications can have side effects, but not everyone is bothered by them or even experiences them. Some go away soon after you start the medication. Your medication was prescribed for a reason, so generally, the expected benefit outweighs the risk. However, if the side effects are concerning or so bothersome you want to stop taking the medication, call the prescribing provider. Do not quit taking your prescription suddenly without talking it over with your provider first.

Biguanide

Metformin, which has been on the market in the United States since 1995, is the only biguanide medication currently approved by the FDA. It lowers blood glucose—primarily by decreasing the amount of glucose made by the liver—and improves insulin sensitivity, making insulin work more effectively. Metformin is available in immediate-release and extended-release (XR) pills. Brand names for metformin include the following:

- Glucophage
- Glucophage XR
- Fortamet
- Rioment
- Glumetza

Metformin is recommended by all the major diabetes organizations as the first medication to start in the treatment of type 2 diabetes. Why is that? Metformin is not only an effective drug, it is inexpensive as well. Other advantages are that it doesn't cause weight gain or hypoglycemia like some diabetes medicines, though hypoglycemia can still occur if metformin is combined with medications that can cause low blood glucose.

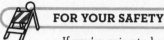 **FOR YOUR SAFETY**

If you're going to have surgery or a procedure that uses a contrast dye, you'll need to stop taking metformin temporarily due to risk of lactic acidosis. Make sure your medical team knows that you take metformin and ask about what precautions are needed before any procedure.

The most common side effects from metformin are the following:

- Gas

- Bloating

- Diarrhea

Luckily, not everyone has these side effects, and when they do, they're usually mild and go away after a while. Another side effect of metformin is it may decrease blood levels of vitamin B_{12} over time. If you've been taking metformin for more than a few years, talk with your medical provider about testing your B_{12} level. Additionally, decreasing insulin resistance through metformin use appears to improve fertility. So women who may have been struggling with infertility or think they are unable to become pregnant may become pregnant after starting metformin. (It is important that blood glucose is in good control prior to pregnancy.)

To reduce the side effects, metformin can be taken with the first bite of food at a meal and started at a lower dose, with a gradual increase. For instance, if your target dose is 1,000 mg twice daily, your dose could be half a pill (500 mg) in the morning with breakfast only for the first few days; you could then add another half dose (500 mg) in the evening with dinner, continuing to progress to the 1,000 mg dose over a week or two. Talk this option over with your medical provider or pharmacist if you're having difficulty tolerating metformin. Another way to decrease the side effects from metformin is by using the extended-release (XR) form, which delivers the medication more slowly throughout the day. But you don't want to cut the XR form in half to split up the dose, because that will release the entire amount at once; therefore, make sure you know which kind you have.

A very rare but serious side effect of metformin is lactic acidosis. If you notice symptoms such as stomach pain; nausea; fast, shallow breathing; general discomfort; muscle pain or cramping; or unusual tiredness or weakness, get emergency medical help right away. Because the risk of lactic acidosis increases with alcohol consumption in conjunction with metformin, don't overdo it when drinking. In general, light to moderate drinking is okay with metformin, but excessive or binge drinking may increase the risk. Talk with your medical provider before drinking alcohol.

Sulfonylureas

Sulfonylurea drugs have been used to treat type 2 diabetes since the 1950s and were the only diabetes pills available to treat type 2 diabetes for a number of years. They work by making the pancreas put out more insulin. Sulfonylurea drugs currently on the market are the following:

- Glyburide (Micronase, Glynase, and Diabeta)

- Glipizide (Glucatrol and Glucatrol XL)

- Glimepiride (Amaryl)

Sulfonylureas have had staying power not only because they're effective at lowering blood glucose, but also because they are available in *generic* form, making them inexpensive as well. Sulfonylureas are taken just before a meal, except regular glipizide, which works best if taken 30 minutes before a meal. Sulfonylureas are usually started at a lower dose and increased as needed.

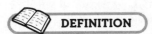 **DEFINITION**

> **Generics** are drugs that are equivalent in dosage and content to brand-name drugs but not marketed under the brand name in order to be lower in cost. Instead, they are referred to by the chemical name. Generics must meet FDA standards to show they are equivalent to the original brand-name drug before they are allowed on the market.

Because of the way they work, sulfonylurea drugs are only effective when the beta cells of the pancreas are still working. So these drugs are used only in people with type 2 diabetes who are still producing insulin.

The most common side effects of sulfonylureas are the following:

- Hypoglycemia

- Weight gain

These medications will continue to trigger the beta cells to release more insulin even if you skip meals or have increased activity and don't need as much. So it's important to have a regular meal schedule and to plan activity to avoid hypoglycemia. Always be prepared by carrying a source of fast-acting carbohydrate with you, like glucose tablets, just in case.

Meglitinides

Meglitinides, otherwise known as glinides, were approved by the FDA in 1997. They are similar to the sulfonylureas because they also cause the pancreas to release more insulin; however, meglitinides are shorter acting. The drugs available in this class are the following:

- Repaglinide (Prandin)

- Nateglinide (Starlix)

Meglitinides are available in generic form, which helps lower the cost of the mediation. Usually, the pills are started with one meal a day and gradually added to more meals. Because they don't work for very long, they are taken just before each meal to help with the rise in blood glucose after eating. If you miss a meal, you don't take the pill.

Like sulfonylureas, the most common side effects of meglitinides are the following:

- Hypoglycemia

- Weight gain

However, compared to sulfonylureas, meglitinides have a lower risk of hypoglycemia. The amount of weight gained is generally not more than a few pounds. If you're just not able to follow a regular meal schedule, meglitinides may be a safer choice than sulfonylureas due to the lower risk of hypoglycemia. It may be difficult though, when you are eating regularly, to remember to take a pill three times a day.

Incretins (DDP-4 Inhibitors)

Incretin-based treatments are available in pill and injectable form. Dipeptidyl peptidase-4 (DPP-4) inhibitors, also known as gliptins, are the pill form. To understand how DPP-4 medications work, a bit of background about what goes on after eating a meal is helpful. Without diabetes, in response to elevated blood glucose following a meal, insulin levels go up and *glucagon* levels go down to help lower the blood glucose. When you have type 2 diabetes, the glucagon level can stay too high after a meal, so the blood glucose doesn't come back down like it should.

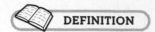 **DEFINITION**

> An **incretin** is a hormone that increases the insulin response after a meal. The two main incretins are glucagon-like peptide-1 (GLP-1) and glucose-dependent insulinotropic polypeptide (GIP). **Glucagon** is made by the alpha cells of the pancreas that regulates glucose production in the liver. To keep blood glucose from going too low, glucagon is released at times when you're not eating, such as overnight.

Glucagon-like peptide-1 (GLP-1) is a hormone made in your gut that tells your brain you're full and slows stomach emptying. Though GLP-1 has a large effect on the pancreas to release insulin and to decrease glucagon, it's only active for a very short time. That's because it's broken down rapidly by the DPP-4 enzyme. The DPP-4 inhibitor medications were developed to block the action of DPP-4 so GLP-1 can stay around longer than normal to help lower glucagon levels and bring the blood glucose level down after the meal.

The first DPP-4 inhibitor was approved by the FDA in 2006. Drugs in this class include the following:

- Sitagliptin (Januvia)

- Saxagliptin (Onglyza)

- Linagliptin (Tradjenta)

- Alogliptin (Nesina)

DPP-4 inhibitors are taken once daily with or without food. The benefits of these medications are that they don't cause weight gain or hypoglycemia. However, they are typically used as an add-on medication rather than the first medication to treat type 2 diabetes. The downside of this class of drugs is the cost; when covered by insurance, the co-pay is higher because they are not available as generics. They are also not as effective in lowering blood glucose as metformin and sulfonylureas.

Reported side effects for DPP-4 inhibitors include the following:

- Upper respiratory and urinary tract infections

- Headaches

Rarely, serious allergic reactions and pancreatitis have occurred in people taking DDP-4 inhibitors (see Chapter 2 for more on pancreatitis).

Alpha-Glucosidase Inhibitors

Alpha-glucosidase inhibitors (AGIs) work by blocking the breakdown of carbohydrates—starches (pasta, bread, potatoes, and rice) and sucrose (table sugar)—after a meal. Their main effect is to decrease high blood glucose related to carbohydrate intake. The two AGIs available are the following:

- Acarbose (Precose)

- Miglitol (Glyset)

AGIs are taken with the first bite of food at each meal to slow down the sharp rise in blood glucose that can happen after eating. The immediate digestion of starches gets delayed, and undigested carbohydrates get moved into the colon. This delay allows the pancreas to catch up and release enough insulin to take care of the meal.

 DIABETES DECODED

Diabetes pills are rarely stopped in favor of another pill. If one isn't getting your blood glucose to goal, another type may be added to the first one. Combination pills are also available for most diabetes medications, which decrease the number of pills you have to take. However, combination pills may be more costly than taking the medications separately.

However, something has to happen to the carbohydrates eventually, and when the colon takes care of them, gas is produced. Therefore, the most common side effects of AGIs are the following:

- Gas

- Bloating

- Diarrhea

These symptoms tend to improve over time, though many people still find the side effects intolerable. To lessen the side effects, AGIs are started at the lowest dose and gradually increased. Following a lower-carbohydrate meal plan also helps lessen side effects. Additionally, while AGIs don't cause hypoglycemia on their own, they may be used in combination with sulfonylureas or insulin, which can cause hypoglycemia. If you are taking an AGI, use glucose in the form of tablets, gel, or liquid; fruit juice; or milk to treat a low blood sugar. Because of how AGIs work, other carbohydrate sources won't be effective in raising your blood glucose.

Thiazolidinediones

Thiazolidinediones (TZDs) , also called glitazones, are known as "insulin sensitizers" because they work primarily by improving insulin sensitivity in muscle and fat tissue. They also decrease glucose production in the liver. The TZDs available are the following:

- Pioglitazone (Actos)

- Rosiglitazone (Avandia)

Of the two, only pioglitazone is available as a generic. In 2010, rosiglitazone came under scrutiny by the FDA due to concern about it increasing the risk of heart attacks. It was not taken off the market, but it was placed in a restricted status. That restriction was removed at the end of 2013 after additional review found the concern was not warranted.

Pioglitazone is taken once a day and rosiglitazone may be prescribed once or twice daily. Neither medication is affected by food, though it's recommended that they be taken with the main meal. Usually, the lowest dose is started and is gradually increased over time. It may take a full 12 weeks to see the effect of TZDs on the blood glucose.

 DID YOU KNOW?

Like metformin, TZDs can improve ovulation in women, making it more likely to get pregnant. Additionally, TZDs interfere with birth control pills, making them less effective.

The side effects associated with taking TZDs are the following:

- Weight gain and fluid retention (particularly if used with insulin)

- Swelling in the ankles and feet

- Osteoporosis and bone fracture

An early drug in this class caused serious liver damage in a small group of people. While this hasn't been the case with the newer TZDs, monitoring of liver enzymes is still recommended. If you're taking a TZD and you have swelling, rapid weight gain, shortness of breath, muscle aches, a yellowish tint to your skin (a sign of jaundice), or unusual fatigue, contact your medical provider.

SGLT2 Inhibitors

There are three FDA approved medications in a new drug class called sodium-glucose cotransporter 2 (SGLT2) inhibitors. They work differently than other type 2 diabetes drugs because they work in the kidneys. Glucose from the blood flows through the kidneys, where it can pass out in the urine or be reabsorbed back into the bloodstream. The SGLT2 in the kidneys is responsible for approximately 90 percent of the glucose reabsorption. The SGLT2 inhibitors block that reabsorption process, and extra glucose goes out in the urine. The SGLT2 inhibitors on the market are the following:

- Canagliflozin (Invokana)

- Dapagliflozin (Farixga)

- Empagliflozin (Jardience)

SGLT2 inhibitors promote weight loss because glucose calories are lost in the urine. SGLT2 inhibitors also don't cause hypoglycemia and may help lower blood pressure.

Because of the extra sugar in the urine, the following are some potential side effects of taking SGLT2 inhibitors:

- Urinary tract infections

- Vaginal yeast infections in women

- Feeling the urge to urinate more frequently

 DIABETES DECODED

Use of SGLT2 inhibitors may lead to "false positive" results for high blood sugar when urine glucose test strips are used for diabetes screenings. If you are a bus driver or commercial truck driver who has to pass a urine glucose test, you need to be aware of this effect.

Noninsulin Injectables

Like the DPP-4 inhibitor medications discussed earlier, GLP-1 agonists are incretin-based medications. GLP-1 agonists are different than DPP-4 inhibitors because rather than blocking the action of an enzyme, they act in a similar way to the incretin hormone GLP-1, which increases insulin response after a meal. Another injectable medication is a synthetic version of the hormone amylin, which also helps to lower blood glucose after meals.

As you have already figured out by the title of this section, the medications listed here have to be taken by injection. These medications have a number of benefits for people with type 2 diabetes but they aren't currently available in pill form due to the way they work in the body. Taking injections can be a drawback, but the benefits may also seem worth it, once you've read about them.

GLP-1 Agonists

GLP-1 agonists works like GLP-1 in your body. As mentioned, the GLP-1 hormone is beneficial in controlling after-meal blood glucose. GLP-1 agonists come in daily-dose and once-weekly-dose forms. The following are the available GLP-1 agonists:

- Exenatide (Byetta and Bydureon)

- Liraglutide (Victoza)

- Albiglutide (Tanzeum)

- Dulaglutide (Trulicity)

DID YOU KNOW?

The discovery of the first GLP-1 agonist, exenatide (Byetta), started out with researching lizard spit—well, more scientifically, the venom found in the saliva of a Gila monster, a lizard native to the Southwest United States. The hormone found in the Gila monster, which was named exendin-4, is similar to GLP-1 but lasts much longer. Exenatide was developed using this research and was approved by the FDA in 2005.

If you have type 2 diabetes and struggle with your weight, a GLP-1 agonist may be a good choice for you. It decreases your appetite and helps you feel full, so you generally eat less while taking these medications. Many people report weight loss, though not everyone has the same results. With many of the diabetes pills leading to weight gain, an effective diabetes treatment that leads to weight loss is a big plus for a number of people.

Exenatide (Byetta) is an injectable medicine that comes in a prefilled pen. One pen is a 30-day supply. Byetta needs to be taken twice daily before meals about six hours apart. Usually it is started at the lower dose for the first month to minimize side effects. Byetta should not be taken after a meal if the dose is missed. If too much is taken or if it is taken at the wrong time, blood glucose may drop quickly, potentially causing severe nausea and vomiting. Bydureon, the other form of exenatide, comes in a single-dose tray or pen that requires mixing (powder with a liquid). For the pen, the mixing of the powder and liquid takes place inside the pen; the tray requires use of a vial and syringe. Bydureon only has to be taken once a week; it doesn't matter what time of day or whether it's taken with or without food. It is recommended to take it on the same day of the week, at a regularly scheduled time, for dosing consistency. The needle size is much larger for the Bydureon than for Byetta, but maybe that's an okay trade-off for weekly instead of twice-daily shots.

Liraglutide (Victoza) comes in a prefilled pen and is injected once daily, anytime during the day. However, it's best to take it on a regular schedule at the same time every day. How long the pen lasts depends on the size of the dose you're prescribed. Like with Byetta, the dose may be started lower to reduce nausea and then increased based on blood glucose results.

Albiglutide (Tanzeum) and dulaglutide (Trulicity), the newest GLP-1 drugs on the market, are each taken as once-weekly injections. Tanzeum, like Bydureon, requires mixing. Tanzeum comes in a pen and the mixing takes place inside the pen. Trulicity also comes in a pen but, unlike the others, doesn't require mixing. The other unique thing about Trulicity is that a needle is integrated into the device, so you don't have to attach one.

The most commonly reported side effect of the GLP-1 agonists is nausea. The other side effects, which are reported less often, are the following:

- Vomiting
- Diarrhea
- Headache
- Dizziness

These side effects tend to diminish over time. If you're prescribed a GLP-1 agonist, you will need instructions on how to take it before starting.

 DIABETES DECODED

If a generic version of a medication you've been prescribed isn't available, the cost is usually quite a bit higher. For brand-name medications, the drug companies may offer discounts for a certain period of time without a co-pay. Check the medication's website or ask your pharmacist about available programs to help cover costs. The companies that make insulin also provide insulin assistance programs for people with financial need.

GLP-1 agonists have also been linked to thyroid tumors in rats, though it's not clear if these medications can affect humans the same way. People who have, or have a family history of, medullary thyroid cancer or multiple endocrine neoplasia syndrome type 2 should not take these medications.

Amylin

Amylin is a hormone that helps insulin work more effectively. Just like insulin, it's made in the beta cells of the pancreas. Since 1987, scientists have been aware that the hormone amylin works alongside insulin to lower blood glucose in response to food. However, natural amylin secretion decreases with damage to the beta cells. The medication pramlintide (Symlin) is a synthetic version of amylin that can be used by people with type 1 diabetes or type 2 diabetes who take insulin to replace the natural amylin they no longer produce. Like the incretin mimetics, pramlintide works to suppress glucagon, delay stomach emptying, and causes fullness, so fewer calories are eaten.

Pramlintide is taken only with meals at the same time as the mealtime insulin. Because you can't mix pramlintide with insulin, this adds another injection with each meal. The following side effects are associated with pramlintide:

- Nausea

- Headache

- Vomiting

- Fatigue

- Loss of appetite

Because pramlintide is taken with insulin, it can increase the risk of hypoglycemia, especially in people with type 1 diabetes. For people with type 2 diabetes, pramlintide is only indicated for use in those taking insulin so precautions are recommended to avoid severe hypoglycemia. The manufacturer states that mealtime insulin should be decreased by 50 percent when starting pramlintide. Frequent blood glucose monitoring and working closely with your medical provider are also needed to ensure safety and to determine the correct insulin dosing when taking this additional medication.

Insulin: The Long and Short of It

There are various types of insulin available, from long-acting to ultra-rapid-acting, with different types having different purposes. Insulin has three main functions to be considered when determining what kind of insulin is needed:

- **Basal or background needs:** This is the amount of insulin required to control your blood glucose for anytime other than when you're eating.

- **Bolus or mealtime insulin:** This takes care of the rise in your blood glucose from a meal.

- **Correction dose:** This is the amount of insulin you need to take if your blood glucose goes too high.

The following table shows the common types of insulin available, as well as their action times.

Types and Action Times of Insulin

Insulin Types	Generic and Brand Name	Onset	Peak Action	Effective Duration
Rapid acting	lispro (Humalog) aspart (Novolog) glulisine (Apidra)	10 to 30 minutes	30 to 90 minutes	3 to 5 hours
Short acting	Regular (Humulin R and Humulin N) U500 regular (Humulin R—concentrated)	30 to 60 minutes 30 to 60 minutes	2 to 4 hours 2 to 4 hours	5 to 8 hours 8 to 10 hours
Intermediate acting	NPH (Humulin N and Novolin N)	90 min to 4 hours	4 to 12 hours	10 to 16 hours
Long acting	glargine (Lantus) detemir (Levemir)	2 to 4 hours	No peak	20 to 24 hours
Combinations (short acting and intermediate acting)	70/30 (70% NPH/30% Regular) 50/50 (50% NPH/50% Regular)	30 to 60 minutes	Dual	10 to 16 hours
Combinations (rapid acting and intermediate acting)	75/25 (75% NPL/25% lispro) 70/30 (70% NPA/30% aspart)	15 to 30 minutes	Dual	10 to 16 hours

Basal Insulin: The Long

Basal insulin is constantly supplied by the pancreas 24 hours a day, 7 days a week, whether you're eating or not. It takes care of the insulin needs other than what is necessary to cover food intake. Basal insulin may be used alone, in combination with diabetes pills, or with mealtime insulin to manage type 2 diabetes, depending on what is needed for adequate blood glucose control.

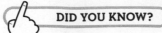

DID YOU KNOW?

Insulin is measured in "units." The most common insulin strength is U-100, meaning there are 100 units of insulin per 1 mL of liquid. Each vial of insulin contains 1,000 units, while most insulin pens contain 300 units of insulin per pen.

Insulin glargine (Lantus) and detemir (Levemir) are long-acting insulins used for the basal insulin needs. They are described as "peakless" insulin, as these long-acting insulins provide a more consistent and flat 24-hour action time. They are usually taken once daily, generally at bedtime. In some people, these drugs don't last the entire 24 hours. If a large dose is required or if it's not lasting the expected time, it is taken twice daily, with the doses approximately 12 hours apart.

There is also one type of intermediate-acting insulin that is used as a basal insulin—neutral protamine Hagedorn (NPH). It is shorter-acting than glargine and detemir, so it needs to be taken twice daily. It is more variable and has a peak action anywhere from 4 to 12 hours after it's taken. It is mainly used during pregnancy or when cost is a factor.

Mealtime Insulin: The Short

At some point, mealtime insulin will likely be required for blood glucose control. Short or rapid-acting insulin is used to cover the rise in blood glucose after eating a meal, which is why these types of insulins are referred to as "mealtime" insulin (also known as nutritional or bolus insulin).

Another use for these insulins is correction dosing, which is often referred to as sliding scale. Unfortunately, sliding scale is frequently prescribed without regard to food intake. The prescription merely tells you how much insulin to take based on a premeal, elevated blood glucose result. For example, if your blood glucose is 151 to 200, you are instructed to take 1 unit of insulin without any additional guidelines on how much insulin to take to cover the amount of carbohydrates in the meal you're about to eat. When used more effectively, the dose to correct the high blood glucose would be added to the mealtime dose and they would be taken together. Correction and mealtime insulin doses should be individualized based on your personal response to insulin and to carbohydrate intake (more on carbohydrates in Chapter 12). Your primary care provider may help you with this or refer you to a specialist who can.

Rapid-acting insulin like lispro (Humalog), aspart (Novolog), and glulisine (Apidra) are the most commonly used mealtime and correction dose insulins. Regular (R) insulin is an older insulin that is still sometimes used, primarily when cost is a factor. Both NPH and regular insulins are lower-cost insulin options if you are on a strict budget. However, they are less predictable in how they work from person to person and even in the same person from day to day, so they are not usually the first choice for insulin therapy.

DIABETES DECODED

If taking a shot before each meal and at bedtime sounds overwhelming, there are some options for taking fewer injections. One way to make insulin dosing easier is to use premixed insulin. With these premixed combinations, the short or rapid-acting insulin is already in the same vial or pen as the long-acting insulin. The convenience of taking only two shots a day does have some drawbacks though. You can't effectively fine-tune doses if you need to adjust just one type of insulin in the mix. You also need to stay on a regular meal schedule to avoid hypoglycemia.

Taking Insulin

When you hear the word *insulin,* probably the first thing you think of is taking a shot. Usually, the picture of the needle that pops up in your head looks literally larger than life, so the thought of taking insulin injections is probably not something you look forward to. However, it is usually much better than what you may have anticipated or dreaded. Most people find injections much less painful than they thought, and are surprised to find out how small the needle actually is.

Unfortunately, a pill form of insulin hasn't been practical to manufacture. An insulin pill would be broken down in the digestive system and become inactive, so it wouldn't do anything for blood glucose control. It's also tough to fine-tune and adjust doses if you're dealing with a pill. However, there are always new developments underway, so you may not have to take shots in the future. A powder form of inhaled insulin has already been approved by the FDA.

Using Smaller or Finer Needles

Needles have become much smaller, shorter, and thinner over the years, to where they are virtually pain free. Pharmacies will often provide the largest needles and syringes available if it's not specified on your prescription. So, when it comes to syringes and needles, it helps to know what to ask for and why.

If you're using syringes to inject insulin, ask your pharmacy for the smallest syringe that's able to hold your largest insulin dose of the day. Syringes come in 30-, 50-, and 100-unit sizes. The 100-unit syringes tend to be the default syringe offered when your dose isn't known. These syringes are marked in 2-unit increments, making an exact dose more difficult. Additionally, the markings are harder to see on these larger syringes because they are closer together. If your largest dose of the day is 15 units, a 30-unit syringe will work just fine. Using the smaller syringe makes it easier to see the markings because each unit is indicated by a line.

To understand needle size, you need to know both the length and the gauge. Gauge is used to describe the thickness of the needle—the higher the number, the thinner the needle. Insulin needles range from 4 mm up to $^1/_2$ inch (12.7 mm) in length and from 32 to 28 gauges in thickness. So the largest insulin needle would be $^1/_2$ inch long and 28 gauges in thickness. For comparison, consider the needle used for a flu shot or other vaccines; even the largest insulin needle is about one third the length and less than half the thickness of that needle, and others are even smaller and finer than that.

If you're using an insulin vial and syringe, there may be advantages to using a 28- or 29-gauge needle. The thicker needles go through the stopper on the vial more easily and are less likely to bend. This is particularly helpful if your hands are shaky or you need more stability. For most people, a 30-gauge, $^5/_{16}$-inch (8 mm) or "short" needle works well. The shortest needles (6 mm, 5 mm, and 4 mm), while potentially the most comfortable, can only be used with insulin pens, because they're not long enough to go through the stopper and draw up insulin from a vial.

If syringe or pen needle samples are available from your medical provider, you can try a few different needle sizes to see what you think. A diabetes educator can also help you figure out the best option for you. Injection techniques may vary depending on the needle length, as well as your body type, injection site, and whether you use an insulin syringe or insulin pen.

DIABETES DECODED

Using syringes or pen needles more than once is not recommended. Because of how thin they are and the way newer needles are made, they won't be as comfortable when reused. Therefore, it's important to dispose of used needles the right way. You shouldn't just throw them in the trash. Your city may have specific guidelines about disposal. "Sharps" containers for needle disposal may also be available for purchase at local pharmacies or drug stores. Check to see if your community has a drop-off site to dispose of the container. For more information, go to safeneedledisposal.org.

Insulin Pens

Many people like the convenience of an insulin pen. With insulin pens, you don't have to go through all of the steps of drawing up the insulin from a vial. Plus, when you're on the go, it is more practical and discreet to use an insulin pen. The cartridge holding the insulin is inside the pen; after the insulin in the cartridge is used, the disposable pen is thrown away. For each injection, a new pen needle needs to be attached to the pen. Another benefit of insulin pens includes the ease of dialing up a dose. If your vision is not so great, it can be difficult reading the marks on a syringe. The pens show actual numbers, so it is easier to tell how many units you're taking. Many pens have an audible click for each unit as well.

Insulin pens are generally more expensive than using a vial and syringe. Some insurance plans don't cover the pens at all, and some will charge you a higher co-pay. Look for discounts and coupons that are available through the manufacturers.

Learning from Past Failures: Inhaled Insulin

In January 2006, the FDA approved an inhaled insulin called Exubera. If you've never heard of Exubera or didn't know an inhaled insulin ever existed, it's not surprising. The main reason not many people know about it is that it didn't sell very well and the manufacturer pulled it off the market a year later. Why did this product fail? Well, partly because as mentioned, insulin injections with smaller needles and insulin pens are easier to tolerate and to take with you on the go. The device to take Exubera was anything but inconspicuous. Folded, it was the size of "an eyeglasses case" (according to the marketing department), but unfolded for use, it was double that size. It was also difficult to get the dosing right and was difficult to use. This led to other manufacturers halting development on similar products soon after Exubera left the market.

However, inhaled insulin has become an attractive option again, with a device that's smaller, less conspicuous, and easier to use. Afrezza, newly approved by the FDA, became available in 2015. Ultra-rapid acting, it starts working just a few minutes after you take it and is gone from your system a few hours later. It can replace an injectable mealtime insulin, but not the long-acting basal insulin. The powdered insulin is available in two doses—4-unit and 8-unit cartridges. The cartridges—each good for one use only—are loaded into a device that is about the size of a whistle. The device dispenses a powdered form of insulin that is taken in through your mouth and then absorbed by your lungs. The following table lists the details about this form of insulin.

Inhaled Insulin

Insulin Type	Generic and Brand Name	Onset	Peak Action	Effective Duration
Ultra-rapid acting	Powder form of regular insulin (Afrezza)	1 to 2 minutes	15 to 20 minutes	2 to 2.5 hours

The most common side effects with Afrezza use are the following:

- Hypoglycemia

- Cough

- Throat irritation or pain

One drawback of using Afrezza is if your dose is larger than 8 units, you'll have to use multiple cartridges. Afrezza will also carry a warning that it may cause bronchospasm—a sudden tightening of muscles around the airways. Cost will also be a factor initially, as insurance companies are slower to adopt new products.

Up-and-Coming Medication Options for Diabetes Treatment

According to a 2014 report by the Pharmaceutical Research and Manufacturers of America (PhRMA), 180 drugs are in development to treat diabetes and related conditions. For example, research is underway for type 2 diabetes treatment that uses a "gut sensory modulator" to deliver delayed-release metformin directly to the stomach. The idea is that it could minimize the risk of lactic acidosis for people with kidney disease. There are also drugs being studied to help treat the nerve damage and pain caused by diabetic neuropathy and kidney damage from diabetic nephropathy.

Several other medications that aren't really new have more recently been considered to help treat type 2 diabetes. Colesevelam (Welchol) is a cholesterol medication that also lowers blood glucose, though the way it reduces blood glucose is not fully understood. Bromocriptine (Cycloset) has been used to treat Parkinson's disease by increasing dopamine levels in the blood. Dopamine sends communication signals between nerve cells and the brain. How the increased dopamine levels work to control blood glucose levels is not fully understood, though it results in lower blood glucose after meals by decreasing the amount of glucose produced by the liver in people with type 2 diabetes.

New diabetes medication treatments are becoming available at an increasing rate. Who knows? You may benefit from a brand-new treatment a year or two from now that's currently being studied in a clinical trial.

Pumping It Up

It can be a bit of a hassle to take mealtime insulin in a public place. What if you could take it without an insulin syringe or pen (or even an inhaler)? An insulin pump allows you to do just that. Insulin pumps are small (about the size of a small cell phone), computerized devices that deliver insulin to mimic a pancreas. With most pumps, a tiny catheter is inserted under the skin and a thin tubing go goes from the pump to the infusion site to deliver the insulin. With a few pushes of a button, you can deliver insulin to cover your meal. Plus, an ongoing dose of basal insulin is delivered throughout the day, like it would be with a fully functioning pancreas.

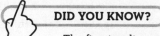

DID YOU KNOW?

The first insulin pump developed in the 1960s was the size of a large backpack. The first commercially available insulin pump came out in 1977 and was not-so-affectionately dubbed the "big blue brick" because of its color and size.

You'll need to change the site and the infusion set every two to three days. A unique feature of one pump is that the insulin reservoir is attached directly to the skin with a sticky backing; this is known as a patch pump. A separate device wirelessly communicates with the reservoir or "pod." To start insulin delivery, you push a button that tells the pod to automatically insert the cannula (a very thin, hollow tube) under the skin, which then stays in place during the use of the pod.

Only rapid-acting or short-acting insulin is used in insulin pumps; you still have to test your blood glucose at least four times a day and direct the pump to give you the right amount of insulin. But new pump systems that "think like a pancreas" are in the works.

Is Pumping the Right Option for You?

If you're currently taking multiple daily insulin injections, an insulin pump may be a great idea. Insulin pumps give you flexibility with your schedule, allowing you to have varied eating times or to sleep in without fear of hypoglycemia, and adding activity without needing to eat a snack so you don't go too low. You can adjust your basal rate based on the time of day or reduce it temporarily for unplanned exercise. Pumps can also allow you to have improved blood glucose control with less insulin. And with less insulin, there's less weight gain.

However, one drawback of pump therapy includes being attached to something all the time. It is sometimes difficult to wear the pump comfortably, especially for women. For instance, where do you put the pump when wearing that little black dress? While there are many creative solutions, you may not want to be bothered with it. And with some activities, like contact sports, insulin pumps aren't as practical.

Also, if you're on diabetes pills and one shot of basal insulin a day, an insulin pump isn't a good option for you. Plus, diabetic ketoacidosis can also happen more quickly with a pump than with injections because only rapid or short-acting insulin is used. You also have to be reasonably comfortable with technology to use a pump.

Last but not least, pumps can be expensive. Without adequate insurance coverage, a pump may be too costly. The pumps themselves have a significant start-up cost, in addition to the ongoing supplies needed, so it can be much more expensive than insulin injections. If you're not getting the answers you need from your insurance company, a representative from the pump manufacturer is usually willing to talk to the company on your behalf to help come up with a solution.

If you're not sure an insulin pump is right for you but you're interested in finding out what it's like to wear one, you may be able to borrow (or rent) a loaner pump to try it out. Ask your medical provider if it can be arranged.

Focusing on Features

There are a number of insulin pump features that may make you prefer one pump over another. You can find everything from simple, easy-to-use pumps with few options to pumps with coordinating continuous glucose sensors (more on this in Chapter 11) and blood glucose meters that download results to the insulin pump at the other end.

If you're considering starting an insulin pump, it's a good idea to contact your insurance company to make sure you have coverage. If you do, your insurance plan may have a contract with a specific pump company, limiting your choice. Additional selection considerations include the following:

- Ease of use
- Visibility of the screen
- Programming options
- Safety alerts and alarms
- Waterproofing
- Ease of getting pump supplies
- Customer support
- Training and education available

And if you need larger doses of insulin, it's important to know the amount of insulin the *reservoir* holds. Some pumps allow for a larger amount of insulin in the reservoir than others, with the largest-capacity reservoirs around 300 units (though larger ones may be coming soon).

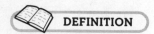 **DEFINITION**

> The **reservoir** is the part of an insulin pump that holds the supply of insulin—usually the amount for two to three days.

A type of insulin delivery option that has some of the features of a pump but lacks the batteries, programming, or computerized components is a no-frills "patch pump." This device has a preset amount of basal and bolus (mealtime insulin) that can be delivered in a 24-hour period. There are only four buttons—one to insert the needle into the skin when the patch is attached, one to release the needle to remove the device, and two buttons (instead of just one, as a safeguard) that need to be pushed to deliver the mealtime insulin. This lower-cost option may be useful for people with type 2 diabetes who don't need a lot of adjustment to their basal rates but are tired of taking multiple daily injections.

As you can see, there are a number of factors in deciding on an insulin pump. Diabetes educators who specialize in insulin pump training are a great resource to help you sort through the pros and cons of the various pumps and to help you choose the right one for you. Ask your medical provider for a referral.

The Least You Need to Know

- Diabetes medications and insulin are often needed to achieve good blood glucose control in type 2 diabetes.
- Diabetes medications work in various ways to approach the different causes of blood glucose elevation in type 2 diabetes.
- Options for types of insulin and insulin delivery may help you avoid fears you might have of taking insulin and provide ways to take it that better fit your needs.

Monitoring—
Putting It All Together

In order to make changes to improve your diabetes control, you not only need to make better health choices, you also need to know what's happening with your blood glucose. Self-testing, or monitoring, your own blood glucose allows you to be able to find out in-the-moment results. Knowing what's going on helps you identify and make changes as needed.

This chapter shares information on blood glucose monitoring, including how to select the right blood glucose meter, how to complete an accurate test, and how to decipher your results to take the appropriate action toward better diabetes management.

In This Chapter

- The importance of testing your blood glucose
- Choosing a blood glucose meter
- Alternative testing sites
- Numbers to track for your diabetes management

Why You Should Test Your Blood Glucose

Monitoring your blood glucose may help improve diabetes control, but only if you do something with the information you receive. While knowing your blood glucose level can alert you to problems and identify opportunities for improvement, if you just test and go on about your day, nothing changes. In fact, because people aren't often sure about what to do with the numbers, this has led some health-care providers to skip the recommendation to test for patients with type 2 diabetes who are not taking insulin. However, if you understand why it should be done, you'll be able to put the information to good use.

When It Should Be Tested

One of the first steps to making testing work for you is learning what the results can tell you. For instance, when you test before a meal, you get different information than when you test after a meal. So when should you test? That depends on what you want to find out.

Primary care providers often recommend that people with diabetes test the first blood sugar of the day right when they get up. This is referred to as a *fasting blood glucose*. Fasting results are used to determine if diabetes medications or insulin doses need to be adjusted. This test, when performed at a lab, is also used to diagnose diabetes.

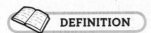 **DEFINITION**

A **fasting blood glucose** is the amount of glucose in the blood after not eating for at least eight hours (usually overnight).

Another time to test your blood glucose is around mealtimes. If you want to know the effect of the food you just ate on your blood glucose, you would test just before and then again two hours after starting the meal. Blood glucose may be higher after a meal, so targets are based on before-meal and after-meal values. Individual targets can vary based on your diabetes goals and health status, so check with your medical provider or your diabetes care team to see what's right for you.

The American Diabetes Association recommends the following blood glucose targets:

- **Before a meal and fasting:** 80 to 130 mg/dL
- **One to two hours after starting a meal:** Less than 180 mg/dL

A blood sugar result of 140 mg/dL or less two hours after a meal is generally considered "normal." If your blood sugar is too high or too low before the meal, your after-meal result may be different even when eating the same type and amount of food. If you take insulin with your meals, it is important to check your blood glucose before the meal and prior to taking your mealtime insulin in case you need to adjust your dose based on the result.

Staying in the Target Range

While you shouldn't expect perfection with blood glucose control, for most people it is generally best to aim for as near normal as possible. Throughout the day, your blood glucose will vary. If the variation is all within the target range, you are maintaining excellent blood glucose control. Sometimes, though, it may also be too high, and sometimes it may be too low. Asking yourself a few questions about what occurred prior to the out-of-range result can help you figure out why it is too high or too low.

Remember, it's not always just about what you ate. There are multiple contributors to high blood glucose, including stress, depression, infection, and lack of sleep. Similarly, hypoglycemia may be related to missing a meal, but increased physical activity, too much diabetes medication, or insulin can also be the culprits. So consider all options when trying to pinpoint times when it's too high or low.

When you experience high or low blood glucose, there is often something you can think of that may "explain" the number, though it may not always be what you think of first. Sometimes there will be one high number that just can't be figured out. It is okay to scratch your head and say "Hmm, just can't explain that one." When there are patterns or trends, however, they need to be dealt with.

One way to help you identify patterns, trends, and contributors to high and low blood glucose results is keeping a blood glucose record like the following. With a blood glucose record, you can not only keep track of your results, but also make notes about why your blood glucose may not be in the normal range for reference.

Sample Blood Glucose Record

		Before Breakfast	After Breakfast (2 hours)	Before Lunch	After Lunch (2 hours)	Before Dinner	After Dinner (2 hours)
Date	Results	106	205		133		
	Time	7:30 a.m.	9:30 a.m.		2:00 p.m.		
	Notes		large bagel for breakfast				

If you'd like to find some different ways to record your results, the CDC has different types of records and log sheets available free for download at cdc.gov/diabetes/pdfs/library/tcydrecords.pdf.

DIABETES DECODED

It's important to wash your hands before testing your blood glucose to improve accuracy. If you've recently handled fruit, for instance, residue on your hands can significantly affect the result. Even hand lotion may impact the result. Using an alcohol wipe is okay when a sink isn't available, but it's not as effective as washing with soap and water.

Things to Consider When Choosing a Blood Glucose Meter

A blood glucose meter is used to self-monitor your blood sugar. These meters are small handheld devices that measure your blood glucose and then display the result. While there are a number of blood glucose meters available with many different features, the basic operation is pretty much the same for most meters. To test your blood glucose, you simply do the following:

1. Put a test strip into the meter.

2. Prick your finger with the lancing device (the lancet is like a small needle) to get a blood drop.

3. Touch the blood drop to the test strip and wait for the results.

The ADA publishes a list of available meters annually in their *Diabetes Forecast* magazine; you can find the 2014 list at diabetesforecast.org/2014/Jan/images/jan14-blood-glucose-meters.pdf. The main considerations when choosing the right blood glucose meter for you are the accuracy, the cost, and the size of the blood sample needed for an accurate test.

Accuracy

Most people say accuracy is the most important factor when choosing a meter. For practical reasons—mainly the high cost of the technology—standards for home meters can't be exactly the same as when your blood is measured at a laboratory. So the accuracy of a meter is based on comparisons to a laboratory reference value.

In 2013, the International Organization for Standardization (ISO) updated their standards for home blood glucose meters to reflect increased accuracy. The current recommended standards state that 95 percent of blood glucose results less than 100 mg/dL have to be within 15 points of the reference value, and blood glucose results at or above 100 mg/dL must be within 15 percent of the reference value. For example, a lab reading of 90 can't show a result less than 75 or more than 105 on your meter, and a lab reading of 130 can't be more than 149 or less than 110 on your meter.

DID YOU KNOW?

The FDA, which regulates blood glucose meters in the United States, has a draft proposal to further increase the accuracy standards.

When choosing a meter, you'll find that the major blood glucose meter manufacturers have been quick to respond to the updated accuracy standards. Companies such as Abbott Diabetes Care, Bayer, LifeScan, and Roche have long track records of providing quality blood glucose meters. However, off-brand meters generally sold at lower cost, which may not have been meeting the previous standards, are unlikely to meet the newer, stricter standards.

If the results from your meter aren't reflecting what you think should be there or you're receiving error messages, there may be an issue with your meter or the way you are testing. Sometimes it just takes a bit of troubleshooting to figure out what's going on. There are some common factors that can influence the accuracy of your blood glucose readings, such as the following:

- You have out-of-date test strips. Check the expiration date on the vial of test strips you're currently using.

- You have improperly stored your meter or test strips. They're sensitive to light, moisture, and heat, so it's important to keep the lid on the test strip container closed and your meter out of direct sunlight. Store them in a cool, dry location.

- You've performed the test incorrectly. For example, you didn't get enough blood for the test or didn't have clean, dry hands.

- Low hematocrit (blood cell) level, caused by anemia or other conditions, can give false high results. Meters have different hematocrit ranges, so you'll need to check for your particular meter.

- High altitude, depending on the type of test strip, can either over- or underestimate blood glucose result. Meters have different altitude limits, so you'll need to check your particular meter information.

The manual that comes with your meter can provide you with the information about the appropriate storage, cleaning, and other factors (such as altitude and hematocrit range) that may affect your results. If you can't find the information, most meters have a toll-free customer service phone number on the back that you can call with questions.

> **DID YOU KNOW?**
>
> It's easier to get a blood sample when your hands are warm, as this increases blood circulation. A good way to increase warmth is by washing your hands in warm water prior to your test. Just make sure they're dry before you poke your finger. Another way to get a blood sample more easily is to hold your hand lower to get more blood flow.

Cost

Do you want to just keep it simple and just know your blood glucose results without other information getting in your way? Or would you like to be able track and trend data by marking which results are before meals, after meals, or after exercise and then download the results into a spreadsheet? Meters range from the simple type that just give results and maintain them in the meter memory to ones with all the bells and whistles.

There are more complex meters available in which you can enter insulin doses, mark events, and even share the information directly with your insulin pump. If having a meter that can be plugged into your computer via a USB port is important, there's a meter for that, too. The following are some other special features you might be interested in when choosing a meter that goes beyond the basics:

• Audio capability or "talking meters" for the visually impaired

• Wireless Bluetooth capability

• Backlighting for easy viewing in dark settings

• Blood glucose averages for 7, 14, and 30 days

• Software that assists with identifying a pattern of results

However, even if you decide on a meter without all the bells and whistles, test strips are still a big cost consideration. Many test strips cost more than a dollar a piece; according to the ADA, current test strip prices range from 18¢ to $1.76 per strip. Sometimes you get what you pay for with the cheaper, off-brand test strips, which is poor accuracy. But less expensive does not necessarily mean less accurate. Each meter has particular test strips designed for it, so you can't just pick a cheaper strip to use. Because you have to use a new strip each time you test, the costs can add up quickly.

Traditional Medicare part B covers blood glucose test strips; though there are limitations on how many, you aren't restricted as to which brand you use. Most insurance companies have preferred brands, so you'll pay a lower co-pay on the test strips with a particular brand they contract with. If you decide to buy test strips through a mail-order company, don't let them switch brands on you if you haven't requested it. To make sure you get the brand you want, you may have to go to a local pharmacy for your test strips. Also, don't let your insurance company or the company you're buying your test strips through convince you to buy a generic meter. While these meters have a lower cost, they may not only be less accurate, they also may not be useful for your provider, because they can't be downloaded to a computer for analysis.

Size of Blood Sample

If the only thing that matters to you is the smallest drop of blood possible, you can certainly choose a meter based on that. In 2014, the smallest blood glucose sample needed for any meter is .3 microliters (mcl), or barely the size of the head of a pin. On the other end of the spectrum, the largest sample size needed for a meter currently on the market is 1.5 mcl. Even at five times larger than the smallest sample, it's still not a very big drop of blood! However, if you have difficulty getting a larger drop of blood, a meter that uses a smaller sample size may be best for you.

 DIABETES DECODED

If you're not sure which meter might be right for you, ask your medical provider or request a referral to a diabetes educator. Helping you select the right meter is just one of the many things a diabetes educator can do.

Is Finger Poking Necessary?

You've probably seen advertisements on TV promoting blood glucose meters that don't require you to poke your finger. When you hear these advertisements, it sounds like you don't even need to get a blood sample at all! Well, unfortunately, if you're not pricking your finger to get a blood sample, you have to get a blood sample somehow. That means choosing another test site. While not all meters accommodate other testing sites, quite a few do, and there is always something in development. Plus, research is ongoing for devices that check glucose without having to get a blood sample, meaning someday, finger sticks really will be obsolete.

Now Featuring Alternate Site Testing

Many meters are now able to accept blood glucose samples from test sites other than your fingertips, such as the palm of your hand, your forearm, or your upper arm. This is called *alternate site testing.* Appropriate alternate sites are listed in the user manual that comes with your meter. Some people find these alternate sites less painful than poking their fingers.

To experience less pain, the clear cap for your lancing device should only be used for alternate sites, while the cap that is the same color as the lancing device is used for your fingertips. The clear caps have a larger hole in the top; while these caps can be painful for taking a sample from your fingertip, it's ideal and less painful for getting enough of a blood sample from alternate sites.

However, there are some limitations if you plan to use alternate site testing. Because the fingertips reflect the most current blood glucose value, the alternate sites shouldn't be used when your blood glucose might be changing. For instance, you should use only your fingertips for testing after a meal, after exercise, if you've recently taken insulin, or when you suspect hypoglycemia to make sure it's an accurate result. The fingertips are still the "gold standard" for blood glucose testing.

DIABETES DECODED

Pricking your finger to the side of your fingertip hurts less because there are fewer nerve endings than at the very tip of your fingers.

Will There Ever Be Another Way to Test?

There are a number of glucose testing methods currently being studied that could make any type of poke or stick a thing of the past. The iQuickIt Saliva Analyzer is one such technology currently in the development stage. It's a small handheld device that promises "easy, accurate, noninvasive, pain-free glucose testing." The description of how to complete the test from the company's website states there is a onetime use "Draw Wick" that you put in your mouth to collect a saliva sample. The wick is then inserted into the device and you can read the result and send it in "real time" to other smart devices like a cell phone.

Another method of glucose testing that's in the works sounds straight out of a science fiction novel—the Google smart contact lens. Google has a prototype lens that can measure the glucose in your tears once every second via wireless technology. While this is not yet ready for prime-time, it sure sounds intriguing.

Another product that has pain-free potential is the GlucoTrack. The company's website states the "GlucoTrack uses ultrasonic, electromagnetic and thermal technologies to noninvasively measure glucose levels in the blood." It does this by attaching a clip to your earlobe that communicates with a device approximately the size of a cell phone. It can store up to 1,000 glucose results for up to three users, as long as each user has a personal earlobe clip.

Yet another way of monitoring your diabetes control is by using a continuous glucose monitoring (CGM) system. This uses a tiny sensor that is inserted under the skin to measure glucose levels in the fluid surrounding the cells, called *interstitial fluid*. Once it's inserted, the sensor can stay in place for three to seven days depending on which type it is. After that, it's discarded and a new one is inserted. A transmitter sends the glucose results through radio waves from the sensor to a small wireless monitor or to an insulin pump with CGM capability. The CGM systems currently on the market in the United States still require blood glucose monitoring at least several times a day. The system needs to be matched up, or calibrated, to a blood glucose meter to improve accuracy.

CGM allows you to really know what's going on with your glucose throughout the day, so you can identify patterns and trends that may need correcting. A nice feature of the CGM systems is that they show a trending arrow so you know which direction your blood glucose is headed. For instance, if you have a blood glucose result of 100 and it's trending down, you may want to eat a snack before you go jogging. Knowing this information can help you avoid hypoglycemia. If your blood sugar does go too high or too low, an alarm will sound so you can stop what you're doing and take care of it. This can be especially beneficial for people with hypoglycemia unawareness.

There are a few downsides to CGM. Like most new technology, it's expensive, and not all insurance companies cover CGM. Because of this, it's primarily for people with type 1 diabetes or people with type 2 on multiple daily insulin injections. It can also generate a lot of information, but it's only helpful if you know how to interpret it. To really use it effectively, you'll need training on the device and the reports. It's also something that stays attached to you; if you already use an insulin pump, having to find another site to insert a sensor may not be ideal.

In the not-too-distant future, these and other technologies being explored may just make pain-free, poke-free glucose testing a reality!

Keeping Track of the Bigger Picture: The ABCs of Diabetes Care

When you have diabetes, blood glucose monitoring with your blood glucose meter is a key strategy to maintain good diabetes control. But for the best overall health with diabetes, it doesn't stop there. Keeping track of the bigger picture, which includes heart health, is also important. There are additional numbers and targets to be familiar with. You can remember what they are using the ABCs of diabetes care. You probably thought you already knew your ABCs, didn't you? Well, when it comes to diabetes, there's even more to find out! Keeping tabs on your ABCs and having regular follow-up visits with your medical provider can help you prevent diabetes complications and live a healthy life with diabetes.

A Is for A1C

The A stands for A1C, which is an abbreviation for *hemoglobin* A1C. This number gives a snapshot of your overall diabetes control for the last two to three months. The ADA recommends that A1C should be at or below 7 percent for most people. What does that mean exactly? Well, an A1C of 7 percent is equal to an estimated average blood glucose value of 154 mg/dL. Each 1 percentage point difference on the A1C is equal to approximately 28 points difference in average blood glucose. The following table provides a comparison between A1C and blood glucose; an A1C from 4 to 6 percent is generally considered normal (for someone who doesn't have diabetes).

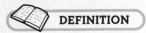 **DEFINITION**

Hemoglobin is a protein found in red blood cells that carries oxygen in your blood.

Comparison of A1C to Estimated Average Blood Glucose

A1C	Estimated Average Blood Glucose
6%	126 mg/dL
7%	154 mg/dL
8%	183 mg/dL
9%	212 mg/dL
10%	240 mg/dL
11%	269 mg/dL
12%	298 mg/dL
13%	326 mg/dL
14%	355 mg/dL

As you learned in Chapter 1, the A1C is determined by a blood test, which measures the amount of sugar attached to your hemoglobin molecules. This test may be done at a lab or even right in your medical provider's office. The lab will draw blood from your arm, but at your provider's office, a finger stick blood sample might be used. You don't need to fast before having your A1C checked.

It's recommended to have your A1C checked about every three to six months, depending on how well your diabetes is being controlled. If you have type 2 diabetes, you're not using insulin, and your blood glucose is in good control, an A1C test twice a year is probably fine. Ask your medical provider how often you should have your A1C checked. If you're not sure what your most recent result is, find out. This number, along with your self–blood glucose monitoring results, gives you a good idea of how well your diabetes care plan is working. As you can see by the previous table, the higher the A1C, the higher the blood glucose. If your A1C is elevated, you need to take some action to bring it down; ask your medical provider what you can do to lower it.

B Is for Blood Pressure

The B in the diabetes ABCs stands for blood pressure. High blood pressure is common with type 2 diabetes, so it's good to know what your blood pressure is and what to do to keep it in target range. Guidelines state that blood pressure should be 140/90 mm/Hg (millimeters of mercury) or lower when you have diabetes. What do the numbers actually mean? The top number is called the *systolic blood pressure*; it indicates the pressure on your arteries when your heart contracts and pushes blood out to your body. The bottom number is the diastolic blood pressure, which indicates the pressure on your arteries when your heart is at rest, between beats. Keeping your blood pressure in control not only helps protect your heart and blood vessels, but it also helps protect your kidneys. Because people with diabetes are more prone to kidney disease, it is critical to keep blood pressure in control to help prevent kidney damage.

What can you do to lower or better control your blood pressure? Eating less salt (sodium) is definitely important (more on sodium in Chapter 14), but that's not the only thing that can help. Eating foods high in potassium—which include fruit, vegetables, whole grains, nuts, seeds, beans, and legumes—is also beneficial. Additional things you can do to achieve better blood pressure include managing stress, being physically active, taking your blood pressure medication as prescribed, and quitting smoking, if you smoke (see the previous chapters in this part for more on these preventive measures).

If your blood pressure is elevated, your medical provider may recommend that you monitor your blood pressure at home to get a better idea of how well it's being managed. If you do check your blood pressure at home, make sure the cuff fits well. There are usually lines on a blood pressure cuff to indicate the range for a proper fit. If it's too small, your blood pressure may be falsely elevated. If the cuff isn't snug enough, it may read your blood pressure lower than it actually is. A wrist cuff may also be an option if you're not getting a good fit. It's important to follow the instructions that come with the monitor to get a good reading, no matter what type you have. You can bring the cuff in to your next medical visit to get a demonstration on how to use it if you're not sure.

C Is for Cholesterol

The last of the ABCs, C, stands for cholesterol. High cholesterol can lead to heart disease, which is more common in people with diabetes. Knowing not only your cholesterol number, but all your *lipid panel* results, can let you know if you need cholesterol-lowering medication. (Strategies for "heart healthy" eating will be covered in Chapter 14.)

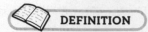 DEFINITION

> A **lipid panel** is a lab test that measures the amount of cholesterol and triglycerides in your blood. Cholesterol is a waxlike substance that your body needs to function. Triglycerides are blood fats.

A lipid panel measures the following:

- **Total cholesterol:** This is a sum of your blood's cholesterol content, which includes HDL and LDL cholesterol. Cholesterol is a waxlike substance your body needs to function. It is made in the liver and found in animal foods such as meat, dairy, and eggs.

- **High-density lipoprotein (HDL) cholesterol:** This "good" cholesterol helps carry "bad" cholesterol out of the arteries back to the liver, making it less likely you'll get clogged arteries. HDL tends to be low in people with diabetes.

- **Low-density lipoprotein (LDL) cholesterol:** Too much "bad" cholesterol in your blood can cause a buildup of fatty deposits (plaques) in your arteries. These plaques can be unstable and rupture, which can lead to a stroke or heart attack.

- **Triglycerides:** These are blood fats. Your body can store excess calories as triglycerides in your fat cells. People with diabetes tend to have higher triglyceride levels. Being overweight, eating too many sweets, drinking too much alcohol, eating too many fatty foods, smoking, being inactive, or having high blood glucose can all contribute to high triglycerides in the blood.

Talk to your medical provider about how often you should have your cholesterol checked and what numbers you should aim for. The ADA recommends the following targets:

LDL cholesterol: Less than 100 mg/dL

HDL cholesterol: Higher than 40 mg/dL for men and 50 mg/dl for women, with 50 mg/dL or higher being better for everyone in terms of reducing the risk of heart disease

Triglycerides: Less than 150 mg/dL

DIABETES DECODED

When you have type 2 diabetes, it's important to have certain routine medical exams and tests done regularly. Your medical provider should check your blood pressure at each visit; check your feet for any problems at each visit, with a more comprehensive foot exam at least once a year; order an A1C test at least twice a year; test your urine and blood to check how your kidneys are working at least once a year; and test your blood lipids once a year.

You should also see your dentist twice a year, go to the eye doctor and have a dilated eye exam once a year, get an annual flu shot, and get a pneumonia shot when indicated.

Source: Centers for Disease Control and Prevention (CDC)

The Least You Need to Know

- Blood glucose monitoring can help you manage your blood glucose if you know what to do with the numbers.
- There are a number of different blood glucose meters with a variety of different features. Some important factors to consider when choosing a meter are accuracy, cost, and size of blood sample required.
- Continuous glucose monitoring offers additional information to determine blood glucose patterns and trends and may help to decrease hypoglycemia.
- You should know your ABCs when it comes to managing your diabetes: A1C, blood pressure, and cholesterol (lipids).

Food as Medicine

Food is such a large and important aspect of people's lives, especially when you have diabetes, so we've dedicated this entire part of the book to it. While making healthful food choices is essential to your well-being, it doesn't stop there when you have diabetes. We cover what healthy eating really means and then take it a step further, explaining how you can use food to help control your blood glucose. We include what to look for when shopping for food, as well as how to read nutrition labels.

In this part, we also share information on how fat and sodium can help protect your heart and lower your blood pressure. We then talk about sugar substitutes, including the difference between low- and no-calorie sweeteners and commons questions about diabetic, dietetic, and sugar-free foods. This part also fills you in on the benefits of whole grains, fiber, and lean protein sources.

Using Food to Help Control Diabetes

When it comes to food and diabetes, most people think they have to get rid of foods—in particular, sugar. Guess what? That's not true! In this chapter, we review the effects of food on your blood glucose and strategies to include the foods you like. We also share tips for smart grocery shopping and ideas for what foods to prepare, as well as how to eat out without going way over on calories and carbs.

In This Chapter

- The effect of carbohydrates, fat, and protein on blood glucose
- Healthy eating strategies
- Grocery shopping for a diabetes meal plan
- Eating out healthfully

How Food Affects Your Blood Sugar

Diabetes meal planning starts with healthy eating principles but also has to take into account how the food choices you make affect your blood glucose. There are three main components of food: carbohydrates, protein, and fat. They are called *macronutrients*, meaning they are nutrients needed in relatively large amounts by your body. All the calories in your food come from these three macronutrients. However, not all foods contain all three macronutrients, and your body needs the right balance of carbohydrate, protein, and fat to help you keep your blood glucose in control.

Carbohydrates

Carbohydrates, also known as *carb* or *carbs,* is the macronutrient that has the biggest effect on your blood glucose. Carbs are broken down by the digestive system into glucose that's used for energy or put into storage for later use.

There are many foods that contain carbohydrates, and they all affect your blood glucose. In fact, the main determinant of an after-meal blood glucose level is the match between your insulin (whether you take it or your pancreas still makes it) and the amount of carbohydrates you eat. If you eat more carbohydrates than you have insulin for, your blood glucose will be too high.

Because glucose is the body's main fuel source, it shouldn't be a goal to eliminate all carbs. Many carbohydrate foods are also good sources of vitamins, minerals, and fiber, all of which are important for your health. Eating the right amount of carbs at the right times is the key to helping you control your blood glucose.

DID YOU KNOW?

You can spot sugars in the ingredient list on a food label by looking for words that end in the letters -ose—for example, sucrose, fructose, lactose, glucose, and galactose. Other common sweeteners include concentrated fruit juice, agave nectar, brown rice syrup, cane juice, evaporated cane juice, honey, corn syrup, high-fructose corn syrup, molasses, and maltodextrin. All of these sweeteners can raise your blood sugar.

Any food with starch or sugar in it contains carbs. Sugars are not just added sugars, but also naturally occurring sugars like the ones found in fruit and milk. For diabetes meal-planning purposes, foods that have a similar effect on blood glucose are grouped together. The carb food groups are as follows:

- **Starches:** Bread, rice, pasta, starchy vegetables (such as corn, peas, potatoes, winter squash, and sweet potatoes), cereal, dried beans, milk and yogurt, fruit, and sweets, desserts, and other carbs

- **Nonstarchy vegetables:** Spinach, broccoli, lettuce, cauliflower, zucchini, radishes, cabbage, and green peppers

Nonstarchy vegetables contain carbs, but much less than the starchy vegetables. Therefore, you can eat quite a bit of the nonstarchy vegetables before they will affect your blood sugar.

When meal planning for diabetes, including quality carbs like whole grains, fruit, vegetables, nonfat or low-fat milk, and yogurt is a good foundation for healthy eating. However, healthy foods can still raise your blood sugar. For instance, if you sat down and ate six slices of whole-wheat bread at one sitting, you would definitely see an effect on your blood glucose! But that doesn't mean whole-wheat bread is bad for you. If you ate the same six slices of whole-wheat bread throughout the day, one slice at a time, you wouldn't see the same blood glucose spike. So how much of these carb foods you eat still counts, whether healthful or not.

Protein

Protein needs to be included as part of a healthy eating plan to provide essential *amino acids* and to build lean muscle mass. When it comes to blood glucose, protein has a much lower effect than carbohydrates. Protein also plays a role in weight management because it tends to help you feel full longer. Including protein foods helps keep you from getting too hungry between meals.

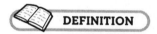 **DEFINITION**

Amino acids are the building blocks of protein. Essential amino acids can't be made by the body and therefore must be consumed through protein foods.

Protein foods include the following:

- Meat (beef, pork, and lamb)
- Fish
- Shellfish
- Poultry
- Cheese
- Eggs
- Plant-based protein foods like tofu, textured vegetable protein, nuts, and seeds

On diabetes food lists, you'll see protein foods listed as meat and meat substitutes, while sometimes plant-based proteins will be listed separately. Meats that are high in saturated fat and sodium like hot dogs, bologna, bacon, and sausage (more on fats and sodium in Chapter 14) can make your blood pressure and cholesterol go up, so lean meats are a better choice for diabetes meal planning. Plant-based proteins are good protein options because they contain heart-healthy fats and fiber. Many plant-based proteins also contain a fair amount of carbohydrates, which should be factored in with other carbohydrate sources in your meal plan. Examples of plant proteins that include carbohydrates are beans (such as kidney, pinto, and black beans and lentils) and vegetarian hamburger substitutes (some brands are higher than others).

Most Americans eat more than enough protein to meet dietary requirements. So how much protein do you really need? Protein needs are calculated based on body weight. Most people need between .8 gram and 1 gram of protein per kilogram body weight per day (g/kg/day). Converted into pounds, that would be .36 grams to .45 grams per pound of body weight per day (g/lb/day).

Here's an example of the daily protein needs for a 150-pound person:

150 (weight in pounds) × 0.36 to .45 = 54 g to 68 g of protein per day

For most people to meet protein requirements, about 5 to 7 ounces of meat or meat substitutes each day will do. The following are some foods that contain 7 g of protein that can contribute to your daily protein needs:

- 1 oz. meat (such as pork, beef, fish, chicken, or turkey)

- 1 egg

- $^1/_4$ cup cottage cheese

- $^1/_4$ cup tuna

Additionally, not all the protein you eat needs to come from meat or dairy. Vegetables and grains also provide some protein, too.

Fat

Words like *crispy, flaky, tender,* and *creamy* are used to describe high-fat foods. Sounds like something mouthwatering and yummy, doesn't it? Fat adds a nice flavor and pleasing texture to food, which is why high-fat foods are so appealing. Does having diabetes mean you have to give up all fatty foods? No, but choosing them less often is a good idea. Fats are, well, fattening.

DIABETES DECODED

Fat has 9 calories per g. One foil-wrapped butter pat at a restaurant is equal to 15 g or 1 tablespoon. That's 135 calories from fat. How many do you use?

You may have heard that fats don't affect your blood glucose. Well, it depends really. Unlike carb foods, you don't often eat foods that are mainly just fat. For example, if you ate a teaspoon of butter by itself, you wouldn't see much of an effect on your blood glucose. On the other hand, a low-fat, high-carb meal like a bowl of cereal with skim milk can cause your blood sugar to rise quickly because it's mainly carbohydrates.

However, high-fat foods are often high in carbohydrates, too. Some examples include deep-dish pizza, fettuccini Alfredo, and cheesecake. These fat-laden, high-carb foods are a different story when it comes to the effect on blood glucose. When you eat foods that are high in both fat and carbohydrates (such as a slice of deep-dish pizza), several things happen. The carbohydrate in the food makes your blood glucose go up. The fat in the food then slows down stomach emptying and delays the absorption of the carbohydrates. This slow-down also delays the rise in your blood glucose, so you may not see a high blood glucose result until hours later. High-fat foods also temporarily raise blood fats (triglycerides), which causes temporary insulin resistance in your liver. The blood sugar will stay higher longer because your body isn't processing the glucose like it should, and your liver gets the message to release even more glucose into the blood. So your blood glucose goes higher with the high-fat meal than if you ate a low-fat version of the same meal. In this case, fat really does have an effect on your blood glucose.

What You Can and Can't Eat

Are you still wondering about what you can and can't eat? The truth is, while nothing's off limits, everything counts! It's all about making smart food choices most of the time. Nobody's perfect or eats only healthy foods all of the time. But you can certainly improve your health and feel better by making nutritious food selections. There is no special "diabetic diet" you need to follow; the recommendations for diabetes meal planning are very similar to the nutrition recommendations for all Americans. So while you don't have to make drastic changes, you'll want to start figuring out your personal blood glucose response to various foods.

"Good" and "Bad" Foods

Making a mental list of "good" and "bad" foods seems pretty easy, doesn't it? You're probably thinking the good foods are the ones that are supposed to be healthy for you, the ones you should eat. The bad foods may seem easy to pinpoint, too—everything you like that you're not supposed to eat! However, the idea of having a good-food and bad-food list (or a can and can't eat list) isn't that helpful to staying on track with your meal-planning efforts. It's human nature to want the "bad" foods more, while the opposite is true of good foods. For instance, you may really enjoy broccoli, but once it's on the list of foods you're supposed to eat, somehow it loses its appeal. So skip the list! Starting with a foundation of healthful foods is still a great idea though.

First, let's discuss what this means. What is healthy eating exactly? Most people know what it's not. For example, it's not skipping breakfast every day; eating fast food for lunch; and snacking on cookies, cake, and ice cream instead of dinner. But what is best for your health and diabetes control?

The Dietary Guidelines for Americans provide some direction about the number of servings of various foods and the type of foods to choose:

- **Vary your veggies:** Consume 3 to 6 servings a day of different vegetables to get various nutrients.

- **Focus on fruit:** Make sure you eat 2 to 3 servings a day of fruit.

- **Go lean with protein:** Get about 5 to 7 ounces a day of lean protein—examples are fish, white-meat chicken, and 95 percent lean ground beef.

- **Choose calcium-rich foods:** Eat about 3 servings a day. One serving is 8 ounces of milk or yogurt or 1.5 ounces of low-fat cheese.

- **Make half of your grains whole**: Consume about 6 to 9 ounces a day, with at least 3 servings whole grains. Examples are 100 percent whole-wheat bread, oatmeal, and brown rice.

 DIABETES DECODED

Eating a variety of different-colored fruits and vegetables helps ensure you're getting the vitamins, minerals, and plant substances you need, because each color is high in different key nutrients. Increasing your intake of nonstarchy veggies is a great place to start because they're packed with nutrients but are low in carbohydrates.

While you don't have to follow the guidelines 100 percent all of the time, these are the basics of healthy eating that set the foundation for your food choices. These guidelines can also help you determine healthy eating goals. If, for instance, you only eat 1 serving of vegetables per day now and the guidelines recommend 3 to 6 servings, you may want to increase your vegetable intake. (Refer to Chapter 17 for ideas to increase your vegetable consumption.)

It's All About Balance

Another way to focus on healthy eating is each meal or each plate at a time. The following figure illustrates how to balance out your plate to keep portions in check using the plate method (choosemyplate.gov; see Chapter 17). Keep in mind, this isn't designed with your particular carbohydrate needs in mind. A registered dietitian (RD or RDN) experienced in diabetes care can work with you to develop an individualized plan.

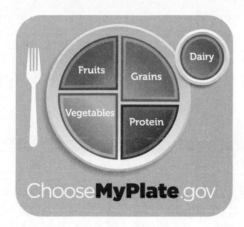

So how can you best balance your plate? The following are some suggestions; take a look and compare your current plate balance to this:

Fruit: Have $^1/_2$ cup canned fruit (packed in juice or water), 1 small piece of fresh fruit, or 2 table-spoons dried fruit.

Vegetables: Consume $^1/_2$ cup cooked or 1 cup raw vegetables. Choose nonstarchy vegetables like broccoli, carrots, spinach, red peppers, onions, and zucchini. If you're hungry, choosing more veggies can help fill you up with minimal effect on your blood glucose.

Grains: Servings vary based on your food choice. Choose brown rice, whole-wheat pasta or bread, or starchy vegetables like a small baked potato or sweet potato. This makes up a quarter of your plate.

Dairy: Have 1 cup of nonfat or low-fat 1-percent milk or 6 ounces nonfat light yogurt.

Protein: Three ounces is generally considered a serving for your plate. Choose lean fish, lean meat, and poultry. If you choose beans or other plant-based protein, you will need to factor in the carbs as part of your total for the meal.

You can also use your hands to estimate how much to eat at a meal. The size of a woman's fist is about 1 cup, though it can vary. Roughly one fist worth of a carbohydrate food equals 30 g of carbohydrate. On average, most people can have 60 g of carbohydrate, or two fists' worth, per meal (more on label reading and carb counting in Chapters 13 and 17). If you're a smaller person, or trying to lose weight, you may only need one fist worth of carbohydrate foods.

For the best balance, one meal would equal the following (the amount of carbohydrates can vary based on which foods you choose):

- Two fists of carbohydrate foods, such as starch, fruit, yogurt, or milk.
- Two fists of nonstarchy vegetables.
- One palm-size protein serving, which is about the size of your palm and the thickness of your little finger.
- One thumb worth of healthy fats (one thumb equals about 1 tablespoon). Olive oil, canola oil, avocado, and oil-based salad dressing, such as balsamic vinaigrette, are examples of healthy fats.

Controlling Your Portions

While you don't have to completely do away with any foods, portions can make a big difference in your success. Smaller versions of not-so-healthy foods fit into your plan much better than large, oversized portions. Another important factor is how often you eat certain foods. For instance, if you eat fast food once a month, you can go ahead and splurge a bit. If you go out for a fast-food lunch five days a week, however, you're going to need to be more careful about your food choices.

 DIABETES DECODED

To get a good idea of how much you currently eat, use measuring cups and spoons to serve up your food. Also, figure out how much your bowls and cups hold. That way, you'll be able to measure the difference as you make changes.

The following table provides a few examples of just how much portions and how often you eat one version over the other can make a difference in calories and carbohydrate intake.

Food Portion Comparison of Calories and Carbohydrates

Large bakery blueberry muffin 610 calories 71 g of carbohydrate	Blueberry muffin from mix 180 calories 27 g of carbohydrate
Big-grab (snack-size) chip bag 400 calories 38 g of carbohydrate	Small bag or 1-oz. portion of chips 160 calories 15 g of carbohydrate
Large bagel 360 calories 70 g of carbohydrate	Mini bagel 120 calories 24 g of carbohydrate

Data source: Calorie King.

The large bagel and the large bakery muffin both have more carbohydrates than most people need for their whole meal! Meanwhile, the calories and carbs in the grab-bag size can easily put you over your recommended amount when eaten with a meal or as a snack. It adds up quickly! However, the portions to the right still give you the same taste and are much easier to fit into your daily meal plan.

Portions, number of servings, and how many calories you need each day depends on your gender (male or female), age, how much you currently weigh, activity level, and height. So if you're a larger, younger, tall, active male, you get to eat the most. However, no matter what size or how active you are, if you're trying to lose weight, you need to decrease the calories you eat and step up the activity from what you're doing now.

Here are a few tips to help you choose smaller portions for your meals:

- Use smaller plates, cups, and bowls.

- Portion out snacks ahead of time. Put individual servings into sandwich bags.

- Measure out leftovers into single portions in small plastic containers and put them in the freezer. They make a great lunch to take to work.

And when it comes to visualizing your portion sizes for your meals, you can use the following markers:

- $^1/_4$ cup is about the size of a golf ball or Ping-Pong ball.

- 1 cup is about the size of a baseball or tennis ball.

- 3 ounces of meat is the size of a deck of cards.

- 1 medium piece of fresh fruit is about the size of a tennis ball.

- 1 teaspoon is equal to the tip of your thumb.

- Two thumbs together is a serving of salad dressing or peanut butter.

DIABETES DECODED

Generally for a snack, women can have about 15 g of carbohydrate, while men can have 30 g of carbohydrate. Most people don't need more than one or two snacks a day. If you like to eat five or six times a day, your meals need to be smaller to account for the calories and carbs in your snacks. If you don't like to snack, that's okay, too.

Making Food Enjoyable

Odds are that you won't follow a meal plan you don't think tastes good. If you're like most people, you tend to eat what you like. Even if you have the best of intentions to change your eating habits, if you can't eat the foods you enjoy, the plan will eventually fail. Plus, you can get bored pretty quickly if you are eating grilled chicken, steamed broccoli, and brown rice most nights of the week. With just a few adjustments, you can make your favorite foods fit more easily into your eating plan, sometimes in tasty new ways. Sounds like a recipe for success!

Healthy Does Not Mean Tasteless

There are many ways to add flavor to food without overdoing the fat, sodium, and carbs. Here are a few flavor tips to choose from:

Curry powder: Curry up your chicken, tofu, vegetables, or just about anything you'd like. Curry powder contains turmeric, which provides the yellow color. Plus, turmeric's active ingredient, curcumin, is a strong antioxidant. So add a teaspoon and spice up your dish.

Low-sodium broth: Sauté vegetables in reduced-sodium chicken or vegetable broth to decrease the fat content. You can use a 1-to-1 ratio—for example, 1 tablespoon of broth for 1 tablespoon of oil, margarine, or butter.

Garlic and onion: These add a nice flavor to a number of foods. If convenience is important for you, keeping a jar of minced garlic on hand and purchasing prediced onions (either fresh or frozen) shortens prep time. Mincing and dicing yourself will save you money though.

Vinegar: If you haven't tried flavored vinegars, there are a number of options. They range from the more familiar cider and red wine vinegars to balsamic, dill, herbal, champagne, raspberry, and more. Vinegar works well in a marinade for meat because the acid helps make lean meat tender. You can also add it to green salads, coleslaw, pasta salad, or a vegetable stir-fry.

Salt-free herb blends: A number of dried herb blends are available without added salt. Some of the flavors include garlic and herb, southwest, citrus herb, and taco. Choose one that sounds good to you and add to fish or chicken, sprinkle on your salad, or include in your steamed veggies.

You can add flavor without fat or carbs, so don't be afraid to experiment and try a new herb or seasoning. If you're already using the previous tips, that's wonderful. If not, pick one of the suggestions and try it out!

Lightening Up Your Favorite Recipes

If you have a favorite recipe that's loaded with fat and calories, you may be able to lighten it up to fit into your meal plan more easily. Because fat increases the calories quickly, lowering the fat content of recipes can make a big difference. The following table shows some substitutions you can make. (See Chapter 17 for more information on decreasing carbs in your recipes.)

DIABETES DECODED

If the recipe is something you only make once a year, it's fine to enjoy as is. However, if you serve it frequently, we recommend making these adjustments.

Substitutions to Lighten Up Your Recipes

Ingredient	Substitution	Type of Recipe
1 whole egg	2 egg whites or ¼ cup egg substitute	Any
Butter, margarine, or oil	Equal amount of puréed fruit (baby-food prunes or pears or applesauce)	Quick breads, muffins, and brownies. For cookies only, substitute only half the fat for fruit
Whole-milk ricotta cheese	Skim milk or fat-free ricotta cheese	Lasagna, casseroles, dips, and desserts
Heavy cream, whole milk, or evaporated milk	Fat-free evaporated milk	Custards, desserts, quiches, and pumpkin pie
Shredded cheese	2-percent-milk or part-skim shredded cheese	Any
Sour cream	Plain Greek yogurt or light sour cream	Dips, casseroles, and desserts

continues

Substitutions to Lighten Up Your Recipes   (continued)

Ingredient	Substitution	Type of Recipe
Bacon	Precooked bacon bits or pieces—decrease amount by half from original recipe	Any recipe calling for crumbled bacon
Mayonnaise	Low-fat mayonnaise	Sandwiches, dips, and dressings
Cream soup	98-percent-fat-free cream soup	Casseroles and vegetable side dishes

Becoming a Savvy Grocery Shopper

Having the right foods on hand to whip up a quick, healthy meal makes a big difference when eating for diabetes management. However, grocery shopping can be an arduous task if you're not sure which foods should go into your cart and which ones should stay on the shelf. This is particularly true if your refrigerator crisper drawer has never been filled with veggies or the entire refrigerator is filled with takeout boxes. Or maybe you know what to get but you're in a food rut with no inspiration or are just tired of being asked "what's for dinner" and you haven't thought that far ahead. Whatever the case, we'd like to share some tips for savvy grocery shopping. With the right knowhow, you won't dread shopping or spend too much time looking for what you need.

Smart Shopping Strategies

Before you even go to the store, make a list. Try to plan ahead for the week and think about what you'll need to prepare meals. Use the nutrition recommendations shared here and what a balanced plate looks like as a guide, making sure to include fruit, vegetables, lean protein, and whole grains. Checking the store ads to see what foods are currently on sale will help with meal planning and save on your budget at the same time. Having a list will help you avoid those last-minute impulse buys and keep you on track. Taking the time when you have it will also help you save time later in both shopping and preparation.

 DIABETES DECODED

See an interesting new fruit or vegetable? Choose one and try it out. The produce manager at your grocery store may be able to provide tips on how to prepare it, or you can check out a number of online resources for what to do.

When you go to the store, focus on the outside loop, otherwise known as the perimeter; this contains many grocery shopping staples. You can find the produce, seafood, and meat counters and the dairy case on the perimeter. (You'll also find the bakery there with some whole-grain options, if you can make it past the donut case.) These areas have different shopping strategies in order to get the best and healthiest options.

The following are ways you can shop smart for fruit and vegetables in the produce section:

- Buy in season as much as possible. When it comes to fresh produce, it's not only the best quality in season, it costs less, too. If it's not in season, purchasing frozen fruit or vegetables may save you money. Frozen produce retains nutritional value, so you're still getting the nutrients you're looking for. Look for frozen vegetables without added sauces or seasoning and frozen fruit with no sugar added.

- Look for produce that's on sale that week in store ads and incorporate those into your menu.

- If canned vegetables or fruit are the best for your budget, rinse them prior to eating them. Rinsing canned vegetables helps lower the sodium, while rinsing the canned fruit helps lower the carbohydrates. Look for fruit canned in its own juice or water packed.

The following are ways you can shop smart for meat, poultry, and fish:

- Choose lean beef, pork, and other meats. Look for the word *round* or *loin* in the name of the cut; cuts like sirloin tip, bottom round, eye of round, and top sirloin filet are lean cuts. Any ground meat that is 95 percent fat free or higher is also lean.

- White-meat chicken or turkey without the skin is lower in fat than dark meat. Because the skin contains most of the fat, buy poultry without skin, or remove the skin at home before cooking.

- Choose more fish. It's a lean protein with heart health benefits. Try fresh or frozen without breading or sauce. Fish, especially salmon, tuna, and mackerel, are high in omega-3 fatty acids. Shellfish is also lean and a good protein choice.

The following are ways you can shop smart in the dairy case:

- Choose fat-free (also called *nonfat*) or 1 percent milk.

- Choose fat-free or light yogurt and sour cream.

- Look for fat-free and reduced-fat cheeses, such as 2-percent-milk cheddar cheese, part-skim-milk mozzarella, and fat-free or low-fat cottage cheese or ricotta cheese.

> **DIABETES DECODED**
>
> If you're not on a tight budget, prewashed, ready-to-go, bagged salads, baby carrots, and other veggies are great timesavers. These handy items can increase your vegetable intake if you typically end up throwing out produce because you didn't have the time to wash and prepare it!

Marketing Tricks to Avoid

You've probably noticed all of the last-minute tempting items like candy, snack foods, and soft drinks. You may have even succumbed to them a time or two. The fact that these tasty treats are staring you right in face is not a coincidence. Marketers are counting on impulse buys to increase revenue, and brands pay top dollar for the prized eye line shelf space. This high investment pays off, as 9 out of 10 shoppers make impulse buys, which means shoppers bought something they didn't plan on buying or need to buy. Plus, it is estimated that women in the United States may consume up to 14,300 calories per year in impulse purchases, and men over 28,000 calories over the same time period.

The key places for impulse-buy products are at grocery store checkout lines and at the end of the aisles. The displays are very eye catching for a reason. They've been designed to be effective and then pretested to make sure they are. These strategically placed items can account for close to 30 percent of total store sales. Now that you know what's behind them, steer clear from those brightly colored displays and say no to the treats at the checkout counter. Stick to your list; you'll be glad you did, for your health and your wallet.

Pantry Must-Haves

Quick meals require not only having a well-stocked refrigerator and freezer, but a well-stocked pantry, too. So what basics should you keep on hand for diabetes-friendly recipes? If you keep your pantry well stocked with the following items, you can always come up with a few easy meal ideas.

Canned Goods:

Applesauce (unsweetened)

Beans, canned (pinto, black, and kidney)

Broth, reduced sodium

Evaporated milk, fat free

Fruit, juice or water packed

Pasta sauce, tomato based

Soup, fat-free cream

Soup, reduced sodium

Tomato paste

Tomato sauce

Tomatoes, lower sodium, diced

Tuna, water packed

Vegetables

Condiments:

Barbecue sauce

Catsup

Cooking spray

Hot sauce

Jam, reduced sugar

Mayonnaise, low fat

Mustard

Oil, olive and canola

Peanut butter

Salad dressing, light

Salsa

Soy sauce, low sodium

Syrup, sugar free

Vinegar

Worcestershire sauce

Dry Goods:

Baking powder

Baking soda

Beans, dried

Cornstarch

Flour

Lentils

Oatmeal

Pasta

Nuts, dry roasted and unsalted

Rice, brown

Sugar

Sugar substitutes

Spices and Herbs:

Allspice

Basil

Chili powder

Cinnamon

Cumin

Garlic powder

Ginger

Herb blends

Nutmeg

Onion powder

Oregano

Rosemary

Paprika

Pepper

Sage

Salt-free seasoning blends

Spice rubs for meat

Thyme

DIABETES DECODED

There are many options for meals with the pantry items. For instance, you can use dried beans and lentils in crockpot recipes; even though they take longer to cook, you can start up your crockpot in the morning and have a meal ready for dinner. Additionally, chili and spaghetti are quick pantry meals. You could even do a stir-fry rice dish to use up any leftover meat and vegetables. A tuna melt on a whole-grain English muffin made with low-fat mayonnaise and 2-percent-milk cheese can also make a quick meal; just add your favorite fruit and veggies to balance it out.

Tips for Eating Out

Most people eat out not only because they like the food at a particular restaurant, but also because they don't have to prepare the food or clean up the mess! However, the more often you eat out, the more you have to come up with ways to fit your choices into your meal plan. The following shows you how to control your portions and make changes to keep your foods not only good but good for you!

Avoiding Portion Distortion at Restaurants

Portions have grown tremendously over the past 30 years. Americans have come to think that huge portions are normal and have begun to expect or even demand them. When choosing a meal, sometimes a smaller portion will work, while other times it's best to just choose another menu item. The following table shows how to swap out some popular items for better proportioned alternatives on the same menu.

Menu Item Comparisons

Original Menu Item	Comparison Menu Item
Burger King Double Whopper with Cheese 1,070 calories 52 g carb 70 g fat	Burger King Whopper Jr. with Cheese 350 calories 28 g carb 21 g fat
McDonald's Quarter Pounder Double with Cheese 750 calories 42 g carb 43 g fat	McDonald's Double Cheeseburger 400 calories 34 g carb 23 g fat

Original Menu Item	Comparison Menu Item
Olive Garden Chicken Parmigiana (dinner) 1,090 calories 79 g carb 49 g fat	Olive Garden Garlic Rosemary Chicken (lighter-fare menu, dinner) 560 calories 32 g carb 21 g fat
Applebee's Three-Cheese Chicken Penne 1,000 calories 91 g carb 46 g fat	Applebee's Bourbon Street Chicken and Shrimp 610 calories 39 g carb 27 g fat

Many restaurants also have lower-calorie or light options available. You should be able to get nutrition information for almost any chain restaurant, though sometimes you'll have to ask. Choose one of the lower-calorie, lighter options or the smaller menu item next time you go to your favorite restaurant.

Another strategy is to order the full-size item but take half your entrée home with you for leftovers. If you plan to do this, ask the waiter to box it up at the beginning of the meal so you're not tempted to eat more than you planned.

 DIABETES DECODED

Focusing on the other reasons you eat out may help you feel like you're getting your money's worth even if you don't get the biggest thing on the menu. That goes for buffets, too!

Special Requests and Other Tips

At restaurants, you don't have as much control over how foods are prepared as you do at home. But that doesn't mean you can't ask questions and find out more information. By gathering information about how foods are prepared and what is served along with it, you can decide what you might want left off or changed.

Here are a few strategies to help you modify restaurant meals to better fit into your meal plan:

Make the menu work for you. More options are now available at restaurants, and more than ever, restaurants are willing to meet special requests. So don't be afraid to ask for sauce on the side, smaller portions, to have meats grilled instead of fried, or to combine several menu items together to get something that fits into your plan.

Be familiar with menu terms that indicate how food is prepared. Terms that usually identify low-fat ingredients include *baked, broiled, grilled, poached, roasted,* or *steamed.* High-fat cooking terms include *fried, crispy, buttered, à la king, alfredo, au gratin, breaded, creamy,* or *en croute.*

Go easy on the sauce. The sauce on an entrée or dressing on a salad can pack on a lot of calories from fat. While requesting these items on the side can significantly reduce fat calories, if you use all of the sauce that's brought to you (which sometimes is more than would normally be included on the dish), there isn't any savings. So add on sauce or dressing sparingly. You can use a teaspoon and measure it out, or use the tines of the fork to dip—not scoop—the dressing.

Skip the bread or chips at the beginning of the meal. If you're with likeminded diners, ask the waiter not to bring any or to just bring one piece of bread with your entrée.

Order first. If you've decided to get the grilled chicken salad with the dressing on the side, great! But if you're out with friends who are all ordering the deep-dish pizza, it's tough to stick with your order by the time the waiter gets to you. Briefly look at the menu, decide, and ask to order first. That way, you'll be more likely to stick with your intended plan. Enjoy the conversation and the company of your friends!

The Least You Need to Know

- Controlling your carbohydrate intake is an effective strategy for blood glucose control.

- There is no one diabetic diet. Healthy eating principles along with carbohydrate control are key strategies for diabetes management.

- Smart grocery shopping and keeping a well-stocked refrigerator, freezer, and pantry can help you stick with a healthful eating plan.

- The more frequently you eat out, the more important it is to use portion control and apply healthful eating strategies to your food choices at restaurants. That way, you can enjoy eating out without overeating.

CHAPTER 13

What Food Labels Are Really Telling You

Most people report reading food labels to make decisions about what foods to purchase. Though many people say they read package labels, when it comes right down to it, most admit that what they're reading isn't always helpful.

In this chapter, we walk you through the Nutrition Facts label, discuss claims about products, review definitions of labeling terms, and more. By learning to figure out exactly what you're getting in a package, you can decide if it's something you want to put into your cart or leave on the shelf.

In This Chapter

- What to know about the front package labeling
- Deciphering claims about nutrients and health
- Reading the Nutrition Facts label
- Differences between serving size and portion size

Front-of-Package Information

Do you ever feel like you're reading an advertisement when you pick up your favorite food package? That's because packages are designed to make you want to buy the product. Many keywords are used to attract you to purchase foods based on current trends. Sometimes statements and strategically listed words can be a bit misleading. Therefore, it's important to not get too caught up in the advertising, nutrient, or health claims on the front of the label.

Advertising

Marketing experts use certain buzzwords to imply that a product is healthy or better for the environment to appeal to buyers. For example, if you saw the terms *gluten free* or *natural*, would it make you more likely to purchase the product? Food manufacturers are counting on it. Let's take a look at different advertising strategies used with each of these terms so you can read between the lines.

DID YOU KNOW?

Many food ads and packages are directed at children, as children tend to want to eat the food with the brand-name package more than the same food in different packaging. For instance, in one study, 75 percent of children preferred french fries in a McDonald's wrapper compared to the same fries in a plain wrapper.

Gluten free: You may find this term added to the label of any food not containing gluten, even when any brand of that product has never contained gluten. With a label of *gluten free* or *naturally gluten free,* brands can appear more unique or special to consumers than others, when in fact they offer the same "benefits" as before. Examples of not-so-healthy gluten-free foods include sodas, chips, and many types of candy.

Natural or **all natural:** Terms like these are used to appeal to the public but don't have a clear meaning as to how that affects the product. In the case of *natural* and *all natural,* they don't have a legal definition recognized by the FDA, so they don't necessarily mean what you think they might mean. However, for many people, the terms *natural* and *organic*—the latter of which *is* defined by the FDA—seem interchangeable, even though they're not. Plus, something that's made from 100 percent cane sugar could be called *natural* and still not be good for you—it's still just sugar.

Even the color of the packaging can influence purchases. For instance, green packaging contributes to the perception that a product is natural or healthy, meaning people looking for healthy alternatives are more likely to pick up a green package. By knowing some of these advertising strategies, you can look past the buzzwords to make an educated purchase.

Nutrient Claims Lingo

Statements on food labels related to nutrient content of foods are regulated by the FDA. Claims about nutrients such as "low" in sodium or "high" in vitamin D are examples of such claims that manufacturers make on food labels. The FDA bases these definitions on "reference amounts customarily consumed," which would be the portion typically eaten, or RACC. While serving sizes on labels take into account the RACC, they're not always the same. The following is a summary of nutrient claims that are defined by the FDA.

Light or **lite:** When present on a label with no additional clarification, it can mean the following:

- The food gets 50 percent or more of its calories from fat. The amount of fat must at least be 50 percent less than the original food.

- The food gets less than 50 percent of its calories from fat. The amount of fat must be reduced at least 50 percent, or the calories must be reduced by one third.

- The entire meal or main dish product (for example, a frozen dinner) is considered to be 50 percent lower in fat than its regular version.

- The food meets the requirements for either "low calorie" or "low fat," and the label needs to state which it is.

 DID YOU KNOW?

The FDA allows foods with a long history of using the word *light* to continue with the use, even when they don't meet the requirements. This includes products such as light corn syrup or light brown sugar. In this case, *light* helps identify the product.

Reduced and **less:** This can be used if there is at least a 25 percent reduction of the nutrient the claim is for—for example, *reduced sodium* or *less fat* than the reference food.

Low calorie: The product contains no more than 40 calories per serving.

Calorie free: The product contains less than 5 calories per serving.

Low fat: The product contains 3 g or less of total fat per serving.

Fat free: The product contains less than .5 g of total fat per serving (can also state *100% fat free*).

% fat free: The product contains 3 g or less of total fat per serving.

Low saturated fat: The product contains 1 g or less of saturated fat, and no more than 15 percent of its calories come from saturated fat per serving.

Saturated fat free: The product contains less than .5 g saturated fat per serving and no more than .5 g of trans fat per serving.

Trans fat free: The product contains less than .5 g of trans fat per serving.

Low cholesterol: The product contains 20 mg or less of cholesterol and 2 g or less of saturated fat per serving.

 DIABETES DECODED

When referring to vitamins and minerals, terms such as *a good source*, *contains*, or *provides* mean the food has at least 10 percent of the daily value per serving. Other terms, such as *high*, *rich*, or *excellent source*, mean the food has at least 20 percent of the daily value per serving.

Cholesterol free: The product contains less than 2 mg of cholesterol and 2 g or less of saturated fat per serving.

Sugar free: The product contains less than .5 g sugars per serving. Sugar is not included as an ingredient.

No added sugars or **without added sugars:** Sugar or sugar-containing ingredients aren't added to the product during processing.

Unsweetened and **no added sweeteners:** The food contains no added sweetener or sugar. The statements must be factual statements—for example, a product that says *100 percent fruit juice with no added sweeteners* on the label must contain exactly that.

Sodium free or **salt free:** The product contains less than 5 mg of sodium per serving.

Very low sodium: The product contains 35 mg or less of sodium per serving.

Low sodium: The product contains 140 mg or less of sodium per serving.

The FDA also allows some synonyms for defined labeling terms. The following are three categories of terms that are considered synonymous:

- Free, zero, no, without, trivial source of, negligible source of, and insignificant source of

- Low, little, few (for calories), contains a small amount of, and low source of

- Reduced and less; lower and fewer (for calories)

While these guidelines are helpful for you as a consumer, they still leave some wiggle room for manufacturers. For instance, according to the FDA, the words *low* or *high* indicate a comparison to another food. The FDA regulates and defines these comparison terms for consistency in labeling.

While it's okay to use a statement that doesn't make a comparison anytime (as long as it just states a fact), if a comparison is implied, it may not be okay to use. For instance, "3 mg of saturated fat" is fine, but "only 3 mg of saturated fat" implies that the food is low in saturated fat, which it's not. In that case, the statement can't be used unless it meets FDA requirements for "low" in saturated fat (1 mg or less per serving).

However, if the manufacturer still wants to use a comparison statement, such as "only 3 mg of saturated fat," they have the option to add a disclosure statement such as "not a low saturated fat food" somewhere on the label. Manufacturers may choose this option hoping you won't see the statement. This disclosure statement is generally not as easy to find as the original nutrient claim, so you have to look for it.

Health Claims

The FDA allows *qualified health claims* for certain nutrients with a strong level of evidence of their potential benefits to state those benefits on labels. In order to use the qualified health claim, both the specific nutrient and the disease need to be included in the statement.

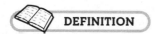 **DEFINITION**

A **qualified health claim** is a claim authorized by the FDA for nutrients that have supporting credible, scientific evidence they may be beneficial for a specific disease or health condition. For example, "calcium may reduce the risk of osteoporosis" is a qualified health claim because it's based on scientific studies.

Some additional health claims that have met FDA requirements and have been authorized for use include soluble fiber from oats related to the risk of heart disease, sugar alcohols not promoting dental cavities, and soy protein related to decreasing the risk for heart disease.

Another type of health claim is the unqualified health claim. These can be claims that aren't necessarily backed by scientific evidence, such as "supports a healthy immune system." These statements are allowed by the FDA on dietary supplements, but not on food package labels. This means a calcium supplement may contain a statement such as "helps promote bone health," while a food high in calcium may not.

Nutrition Facts Label

The iconic Nutrition Facts label was introduced over 20 years ago to help consumers make healthier food choices. The Nutrition Facts label provides a lot of information, but if you know what to look for and how it works, you can make your choices and get in and out of the grocery store more quickly! Let's break down the pieces of a Nutrition Facts label using this sample label.

Nutrition Facts

Serving Size 1/2 cup (63g)
Serving Per Container About 4

Amount Per Serving

Calories 100	Calories from Fat 32	

		% Daily Value*
Total Fat	3.5g	**5%**
Saturated Fat	2g	**10%**
Trans Fat	0g	
Cholesterol	20mg	**0%**
Sodium	45mg	**2%**
Total Carbohydrate	15g	**5%**
Dietary Fiber	0g	**0%**
Sugars	11g	
Protein	3g	

Vitamin A	3%
Vitamin C	0%
Calcium	6%
Iron	0%

*Percent Daily Values are based on a 2,000 calorie diet.
Your daily value may be higher or lower depending on
your calorie needs.

	Calories:	2,000	2,500
Total Fat	Less than	65g	80g
Sat Fat	Less than	20g	25g
Cholesteral	Less than	300mg	300mg
Sodium	Less than	2,400mg	2,400mg
Total Carbohydrate		300g	375g
Dietary Fiber		25g	30g

Serving size: To get the best use of the Nutrition Facts label, always start with this. Serving sizes are listed in volume and by weight in g. The serving size here is $^1/_2$ cup, which weighs 63 g. Weight in g is not really that important unless you're weighing out your food on a scale; normally you'll use the volume measure. Consider how this product fits into your meal plan and health goals. Would you only eat the amount listed as a serving, or would your portion be larger?

Calories: This product contains 100 calories per $^1/_2$-cup serving. Think about your other food choices for the day to decide whether or not this food fits in with your daily calorie target.

Nutrients column: This is where you'll find the nutrients you should limit—total fat, saturated fat, trans fat, and sodium. This label shows there are total fat (3.5 g), saturated fat (2 g), trans fat (0 g), and sodium (45 mg) per serving. This product doesn't contain trans fat, which is good. The sodium content is low, so that's also a plus. Per serving, this product is not high in any of the nutrients you need to limit.

Total carbohydrate: Next is total carbohydrate (15 g), and then dietary fiber (0 g) and sugars (11 g). The total carbohydrate is the most important number here. Notice how the words *total carbohydrate* are in bold and the dietary fiber and sugars are indented and included underneath. Both the dietary fiber and sugars are included in the total carbohydrate amount, so total carbohydrate is all you count. All carbohydrates affect your blood glucose, not just the sugars. You don't have to count sugars at all, because they've already been counted in the total carbohydrate.

Some people subtract the dietary fiber from the total carbohydrate because it's not digested, meaning it shouldn't affect the blood glucose. However, guidelines recommend that only half the dietary fiber would be subtracted from the total carbohydrate and only when the fiber content is above 5 g. If you have type 2 diabetes and you're trying to lose weight, it's better not to subtract any of the fiber—just use the total carbohydrate amount.

 DIABETES DECODED

> The daily value for dietary fiber is 25 g, which is equal to 100 percent of the daily value. This means that you eat "at least" this amount of dietary fiber per day.

Protein: One serving of this product provides 3 g of protein.

Vitamins and beneficial nutrients: Underneath the bold line, you'll see vitamins A and C, calcium, and iron. These are all nutrients you want to make sure you get enough of. The amounts aren't listed—only the percentage of the daily value in one serving.

% daily value: The % daily value is based on a 2,000-calorie diet, so it's comparing everything on the label to the targets based on that calorie intake. Check out the footnote at the bottom of the label showing amounts of each nutrient recommended for 2,000-calorie and 2,500-calorie diets. The amounts listed under the 2,000-calorie column are the ones used to determine the % daily value. You'll see "less than" after the nutrients that need to be limited; the amounts listed after that are considered to be the upper limits for those nutrients.

Even though 2,000 calories may not be your recommended calorie level, the % daily value can still make it easy to do quick comparisons between products before you read the rest of the label. If the % daily value is 5 percent or less, it's low in whatever it's listed next to. If it's 20 percent or higher, it's high in whatever it's listed next to. If you have all greater than 20 percent next to fat, saturated fat, and sodium, you may want to put that product back on the shelf and keep looking! This product is low in total fat (5 percent) and sodium (2 percent), while the saturated fat (10 percent)—though not considered low—can still be worked into your meal plan.

Serving or Portion—What's the Difference?

You may think that serving size and portions are the same thing, but when it comes right down to it, there's an important difference. The serving size on a food label tells you only one thing—the reference amount of the food that the Nutrition Facts food label is based on. So if you eat the amount of food that's shown as the serving size listed on the package, you get the amount of calories, fat, sodium, carbohydrate, and so on listed on the label. There would be no difference from the amount listed compared to what you ate.

However, the serving size isn't necessarily the portion you'll choose to eat. If you choose to eat only half of the listed serving size, you'll only get half the amount of calories, fat, sodium, and carbohydrate listed. Or if you choose to eat double the serving, you know what happens next. The portion you eat determines how many calories and nutrients you actually consume. So the portion size is what you choose, while the serving size is simply what's listed on the label.

When you're reading a Nutrition Facts label, you need to consider if the serving size listed is a reasonable amount and think about the portion you would choose. In order to really know how many calories and nutrients you're getting from a particular food, you need to measure out your own portion and compare it to the serving size listed on the label. Sometimes this can be a real eye-opener; other times it may be the same as the portion you're already eating.

Anytime you choose a different portion than that listed as the serving size, you'll have to do some math to figure out what you're actually getting. For example, let's say from a Nutrition Facts label, you learn the following information (assume the product contains no saturated fat, trans fat, or cholesterol):

Serving Size	1/2 cup
Calories	200
Total Fat	14 g
Sodium	40 mg
Total Carbohydrate	17 g
Dietary Fiber	2 g
Sugars	14 g
Protein	3 g

If you eat 1/2 cup of this product, you've eaten 200 calories, 14 g of fat, 17 g of carbohydrate, and 3 g of protein.

What if your portion is $1^1/_2$ cups? Would it still fit into your meal plan? Because your portion size is 3 times as big as the serving size, you would have to multiply the original amounts by 3 to figure out how much you're actually eating:

Calories: $200 \times 3 = 600$

Total Fat: $14 \times 3 = 42$

Sodium: $40 \times 3 = 120$

Total Carbohydrate: $17 \times 3 = 51$

Protein: $3 \times 3 = 9$

So by eating 3 times the serving size, you get 600 calories, 42 g of fat, 51 g of carbohydrates, and 9 g of protein. That makes a big difference! While the food in the serving size shown may fit into your meal plan with little difficulty, the much larger portion doesn't work as well. You don't have to stick with the serving size on the label, but remember to consider how portions count when buying the food and when deciding how much of it to eat!

Proposed Changes to the Nutrition Facts Label

The FDA is recommending an update to the original Nutrition Facts label to reflect changes based on studies and consumer feedback. If these changes are approved, you will see some noticeable differences, such as the following:

- Calories per serving will be featured much more prominently.

- Because it's currently difficult to figure out whether sugars are naturally occurring or added to a food, there will be an additional line under Total Carbohydrate for added sugars.

- Contents of certain nutrients such as vitamin D and potassium will be listed.

- Vitamins A and C would become voluntary to include on the label.

- The percent daily value for calcium and iron would continue to be listed, but the actual content of these nutrients would be added for clarity.

- Sodium will be updated from 2,400 mg for the reference range to 2,300 mg.

One major change the FDA is also proposing that would be beneficial to consumers is having the serving size recommend to the amounts that people typically eat or drink. For instance, if a bottle of soda is 20 ounces, the serving size would be based on the whole container, not just part of it. The serving size (along with the calories) would be listed in bigger font than the rest of the label content so it stands out at a quick glance. While some serving sizes may actually decrease if the amount typically eaten is less than the current size, most will be larger. Once the serving size on the container reflects a more typical portion, it should be easier to determine the calories and nutrients you'll get from the food. If you're curious, proposed changes can be viewed on the fda. gov website.

The Least You Need to Know

- The front packaging is geared toward getting you to purchase the product. Look at the Nutrition Facts label and ingredient list to find out more before you buy; don't fall for the advertising hype.

- Nutrient content claims and qualified health claims are defined by the FDA. Once you learn the definitions, you gain a better understanding of what the terms are telling you.

- You can use the % daily values on the Nutrition Facts label to quickly determine if the product deserves a closer look. If the % daily value is 5 percent or less, it's low in whatever it's listed next to. If it's 20 percent or higher, it's high in whatever it's listed next to.

- The portion that you actually eat is what counts, not just the amount of the serving size listed on the Nutrition Facts label. You have to count everything you eat.

Fats and Sodium

The American Heart Association (AHA) states that at least 65 percent of people with diabetes die from stroke or heart disease. People with diabetes are at two to four times more risk of getting heart disease than people without diabetes. A crucial factor for your heart health is what you eat, particularly when it comes to saturated fat, trans fat, and sodium intake. By controlling the amount and types of fats and sodium you consume, you can improve your heart health and decrease your risk of heart disease.

In this chapter, we share which fats are heart healthy and which ones increase your risk of heart disease, as well as how reducing sodium is a key strategy in blood pressure control. We also help you understand the information concerning fats and sodium on food labels and recommend a few changes you can make to help lower the unhealthy fats and sodium in your meal plan.

In This Chapter

- Decreasing saturated and trans fats
- Identifying heart-healthy fats
- Lowering your sodium intake

The Basics on Fat

Fats can be added to other foods in the form of oil, margarine, butter, salad dressing, mayonnaise, nut butters, lard, sour cream, cream cheese, and shortening. Fats can also come from plant foods like avocados, nuts, seeds, and olives. When it comes to fats, science can be confusing at times, and headlines can be conflicting. For instance, one minute it sounds like margarine is better, and another minute butter is being touted as the better fat. Plus, spreads can be blended into different combinations—butter with canola oil, margarine made with yogurt, and so on—making it that much more difficult to parse the good from the bad. So where do you start?

To begin, let's take a look at a Nutrition Facts label. The FDA requires that total fat, saturated fat, and trans fat be included on the label for all foods; you can see those circled in our sample label. However, the numbers mean nothing without some context. Here's what you need to pay attention to in order to gain a better understanding of the amount of fat in your food:

Nutrition Facts

Serving Size 2/3 cup (55g)
Serving Per Container About 8

Amount Per Serving

Calories 230 | Calories from Fat 72

% Daily Value*

Total Fat	8g	**12%**
Saturated Fat	1g	**5%**
Trans Fat	0g	
Cholesterol	0mg	**0%**
Sodium	490mg	**20%**
Total Carbohydrate	37g	**12%**
Dietary Fiber	4g	**16%**
Sugars	1g	
Protein	3g	

Vitamin A	10%
Vitamin C	8%
Calcium	20%
Iron	45%

*Percent Daily Values are based on a 2,000 calorie diet. Your daily value may be higher or lower depending on your calorie needs.

	Calories:	2,000	2,500
Total Fat	Less than	65g	80g
Sat Fat	Less than	20g	25g
Cholesteral	Less than	300mg	300mg
Sodium	Less than	2,400mg	2,400mg
Total Carbohydrate		300g	375g
Dietary Fiber		25g	30g

Serving size: This is the amount that all of the label's information is based on. So, for example, if you're comparing two products and they have different serving sizes, you'll have to adjust the serving size of one to match the other to make a fair comparison. In the case of this product, the serving size is $^2/_3$ cup (as indicated by the arrow).

Also, if you choose to eat a different amount than the listed serving size, you'll have to adjust your totals. For instance, if you choose to eat double the serving ($1^1/_3$ cups) of this product, you'll have to double the amount of fat, saturated fat, and trans fat you're tallying up.

Calories: Check to see how many calories are in a serving. This product has 230 calories in each $^2/_3$-cup serving. There are eight $^2/_3$-cup servings in the entire package, so if you ate the whole container you would consume 1,840 calories ($230 \times 8 = 1,840$).

Nutrients column: This tells you the amounts of specific nutrients in each serving. The first section—total fat, saturated fat, trans fat, and cholesterol—are nutrients you want to limit. In order to determine your daily intake of these nutrients, you would need to keep a running total of the g or mg (depending on what you're tracking—for example, total fat or cholesterol) based on the portion sizes you've eaten. It is recommended to keep cholesterol under 300 mg per day, and under 200 mg if you have heart disease.

% daily value column: This gives you the percentage of each nutrient per serving, when a recommended amount is available. At quick glance, you can tell if something is low if the % daily value is 5 percent or less; if it's 20 percent or higher, it's high. This product has 5 percent of the saturated fat for the day in one serving, so it's considered low in saturated fat.

Trimming the Unhealthy Fats

Recommendations to decrease saturated fats and trans fats are based on the fact that intake of these fats raises LDL (bad) cholesterol. Elevated LDL cholesterol contributes to the buildup of fatty deposits in your arteries, which increases the risk for heart attack and stroke. In the late 1980s, a low-fat diet craze started in efforts to lower LDL cholesterol and along with it, heart disease. Since then, it's been determined that there's more to the equation. While lowering the unhealthy fats is still the first step, the food choices you replace it with also matter. Choosing fruits, vegetables, whole grains, and healthy fats in place of foods high in saturated fat and trans fat is the other piece of the nutrition puzzle when it comes to heart health.

Limiting Saturated Fat

Saturated fatty acids are the building blocks of saturated fats. Sources of saturated fat include cheese, meat (particularly high-fat meats such as sausage, bacon, prime rib, rib-eye, and hot dogs), poultry with skin, cream or half and half, milk (low-fat and whole), ice cream, and eggs.

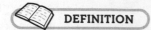

DEFINITION

Saturated fatty acids make up saturated fats. Fatty acids are molecules that are mainly made up of carbon and hydrogen atoms. Carbon atoms in a fatty acid are lined up in a row, like a string of beads. When the maximum amount of hydrogen atoms are attached to every carbon atom, the carbons are "saturated" with hydrogen.

Saturated fats are mainly found in animal foods with a few exceptions, such as coconut oil, palm oil, and palm kernel oil. While both animal- and plant-based fats can be saturated, only animal foods contain cholesterol. You can identify saturated fats because they are solid at room temperature. For instance, a stick of butter is solid even when not refrigerated, whereas vegetable oils are liquid. Coconut oil, also a saturated fat, doesn't really look like oil at all, but rather a thick white paste.

Guidelines vary as to the recommended intake of saturated fat. The Dietary Guidelines for Americans recommend no more than 10 percent of calories per day come from saturated fats; however, the AHA aims to further reduce heart disease by recommending approximately 6 percent of calories from saturated fat.

Due to the increased risk of heart disease for people with diabetes, the AHA's more conservative recommendation is prudent. To meet the AHA target, most women have a recommended intake of 11 to 15 g of saturated fat per day based on a variation in calorie needs; meanwhile, most men have a daily recommendation of 13 to 19 g of saturated fat. However, if you currently include a lot of foods high in saturated fat, you may want to aim for 10 percent of your calories initially, and then gradually decrease.

DID YOU KNOW?

Even though some groups don't agree with the AHA regarding saturated fats, the AHA bases recommendations on evidence over time. They continue to recommend limiting saturated fats to decrease risk of heart disease because the evidence to increase saturated fat is not as compelling as reducing it. Because this recommendation goes along with eating more fruit, vegetables, and whole grains and choosing lean protein and reduced fat or fat-free dairy products, it makes good nutritional sense. Plus, if you replace high-fat foods with these lower-fat options, it can help with your weight-loss efforts.

Get the Trans Outta There

Trans fat is made by partially hydrogenating oil. This type of fat is formed when hydrogen is added to an unsaturated liquid oil, turning it into solid fat. An example of trans fat is vegetable shortening. Shortening is vegetable oil that's been partially hydrogenated, turning it into a solid at room temperature.

Trans fats have historically been used in food products because they're inexpensive and they increase shelf life, stability, and texture of a food product. Now that the health risk of trans fats are recognized, however, many products have been reformulated to remove them. One thing that helped speed up this industry-wide change was the FDA requirement that trans fat content had to be listed on Nutrition Facts labels. The intake of trans fat decreased significantly in the United States due to this label change, and because most restaurants are no longer using oils containing trans fats to fry foods.

However, trans fat can still be found in some of the following foods: cookies; crackers; cakes; refrigerated, ready-to-bake goods like cinnamon rolls and sweet rolls; some brands of microwave popcorn; shortening; and some margarines.

To minimize trans fat in your diet as much as possible, aim for less than 2 g per day. The FDA allows food manufacturers to list "0 g" of trans fat on the label if the product contains less than .5 g per serving, so when examining a product label for your food of choice to see whether it contains any trans fat, look for the words *partially hydrogenated* in the ingredient list. If you find them, there's some trans fat in the product.

More Healthy Fats, Please

Even if you've never heard of monounsaturated fatty acid (MUFA) or polyunsaturated fatty acid (PUFA) before, it's certain you've eaten them. MUFA and PUFA are two types of heart-healthy fats that should be included in your usual eating plan. By replacing foods high in saturated fat and trans fat with foods containing MUFAs and PUFAs, you may be able to lower your risk of heart disease. Plus, many foods that are good sources of MUFA and PUFA also contain other nutrients that are beneficial to your health.

MUFAs

Good sources of MUFA include olive oil, canola oil, avocados, nuts, nut butters, peanut oil, and olives. If you've heard about health benefits from following a Mediterranean diet, inclusion of foods high in MUFAs are one of the reasons it's so healthy (see Chapter 17 for more on the Mediterranean diet).

 DIABETES DECODED

Remember that any source of pure fat, heart healthy or not, contains approximately 45 calories per teaspoon (about the size of the tip of your thumb). Fat calories add up quickly even in small amounts, so unless you want to gain weight, you'll need to keep the total amount of fat in check to avoid overdoing it on the calories.

MUFAs are helpful in reducing LDL (bad) cholesterol and may increase HDL (good) cholesterol, making them especially useful in fighting heart disease. Along with decreasing cholesterol, MUFAs may also benefit insulin levels and blood glucose control. Sounds like a win-win.

PUFAs

Omega-6 and omega-3 fatty acids are types of polyunsaturated fats (PUFAs) that are essential fatty acids, meaning your body can't make them; you have to get them through food. Both omega-3 and omega-6 are very important for many body functions. Omega-6s can be found in most types of vegetable oil, mayonnaise, salad dressings, poultry, beef, pork, and nuts and seeds. Meanwhile, omega-3 fatty acids are the type of polyunsaturated fat that's found in fish (such as salmon, albacore tuna, trout, mackerel, sardines, and herring), with walnuts, flaxseeds, and leafy green vegetables good plant sources for it. Most Americans eat more omega-6 fatty acids than omega-3 fatty acids because the food sources high in omega-6 are more plentiful in the average American eating pattern.

Eating foods high in PUFAS can help decrease your risk of heart disease by lowering your bad cholesterol and triglycerides. PUFAs may also help decrease your risk of developing type 2 diabetes by decreasing insulin resistance. Likely due to their function in the formation of hormones that regulate blood clotting, inflammation, and contraction and relaxation of the arterial walls, omega-3s have been shown to be effective in lowering blood pressure, decreasing the risk of blood clots, protecting against stroke and heart failure, and improving irregular heartbeat.

Both the AHA and the ADA recommend eating two servings of fish per week, especially those high in omega-3s. A serving of fish is 3.5 ounces or about the size of a deck of cards or a checkbook.

 FOR YOUR SAFETY

While increasing omega-3 fatty acids from food sources is better than taking supplements, your medical provider may recommend supplements if you're unable to get enough omega-3s through foods. If that's the case, it's important not to take more than the recommended dose. Doses over 3,000 mg (3 g) may increase the risk of bleeding. If you bruise easily; have a bleeding disorder; or take warfarin (Coumadin), clopidogrel (Plavix), or aspirin, make sure to tell your medical provider.

Increasing Your Intake of MUFAs and PUFAs

MUFAs and PUFAs aren't required to be included on a Nutrition Facts label. However, manufacturers can voluntarily include them. You will usually find them on a label of foods that are good sources of MUFAs and PUFAs, so that's a good place to start. The AHA recommends between 25 and 35 percent of your total calories come from fat. For a 2,000-calorie diet, that would equal 500 calories or 56 g of fat to 700 calories or 78 g of fat. So you'll want to work MUFA and PUFA fats into your total fat intake for the day.

How can you increase your intake of these healthy fats while limiting saturated and trans fats? Here are a few ideas:

- Cook with olive, canola, sunflower, or corn oil instead of butter.

- Choose more fatty fish, shellfish, and poultry without skin in place of high-fat meats or poultry with skin.

- Have a small handful of unsalted nuts or seeds for a snack instead of a candy bar, donut, or other snack food.

- Add a slice of avocado and veggies to an omelet instead of ham and cheese.

- Include ground flaxseeds or walnuts in your oatmeal in the morning in place of a pat of butter.

Remember, if you need to lose weight, extra calories from any source—including MUFAs and PUFAs—can still cause you to gain weight. So you can't just add them to what you currently eat; there has to be a tradeoff. If you want to lose weight, you'll still need to eat fewer calories from all sources than what you're eating now.

Time to Decide: Butter or Margarine?

Now that you've expanded your knowledge of fats, let's consider a common decision people have to make: butter or margarine? The following table provides a comparison of various butter and margarine products (average of brands); take a look and see what choice you would make.

Product Comparison for a One-Tablespoon Serving of Butter and Margarine Spreads

Product	Calories*	Total Fat	Saturated Fat	Trans Fat
Butter	100	11 g	7 g	0 g
Butter, light	70	8 g	5 g	0 g
Butter, light with canola oil	50	5 g	2 g	0 g
Margarine, stick	101	11 g	2 g	1 to 2 g
Margarine, tub	100	11 g	3 g	0 g
Margarine, tub light	45	5 g	1.5 g	0 g
Margarine, tub, light, with yogurt	45	5 g	1.5 g	0 g
Vegan olive oil spread	80	9 g	0 g	0 g

*The products in this table only contain calories from fat and represent an average of brands available on the market.

Would you choose the butter? With 7 g of saturated fat per tablespoon, you could quickly go over the recommended amount for the day! What about the light butter with canola oil blend? It compares pretty favorably and you still get that buttery taste. The vegan (no animal ingredients) spread doesn't provide any saturated or trans fat, so it gets good marks for that. If you're going for the lowest calorie and saturated fat content combined, the light margarines look good.

So what do the experts say? For spreads, a soft tub margarine—typically the lowest in saturated fat, with a liquid oil as the first ingredient, 0 g trans fat, and no partially hydrogenated oils—is the best option. However, for baking, light products like this don't yield a quality baked good. In this case, look for trans-fat-free stick margarine. It reduces saturated fat and still gives baked goods the quality you're looking for.

Reducing Sodium

When you hear the word *sodium,* you probably think salt. While the two words tend to be used like they're the same, actually they're not. Sodium is a component of salt. Table salt is made up of 40 percent sodium and 60 percent chloride by weight, and a teaspoon of table salt provides 2,300 mg of sodium.

> **DID YOU KNOW?**
>
> The difference between sea salt and table salt is not as big as you might think. Both are made up of about 40 percent sodium; however, sea salt is evaporated directly from sea water with minimal processing. So the original minerals contained in the seawater stay in the salt, providing a unique color and flavor. Also, sea salt doesn't usually have iodine added to it. Iodine is needed for your thyroid gland to function normally, so it's added to table salt to prevent thyroid problems due to iodine deficiency.

However, salt is a major source of sodium in the American food supply. Salt helps not only with flavor in food, but also improves texture, inhibits fermentation, and acts as a stabilizer and binder. Salt and ingredients containing sodium are also used to maintain quality and safety; and to lengthen the shelf life of a product by preventing bacteria, mold, and yeast from growing in the food.

About 90 percent of Americans eat more sodium than they should, according to the CDC. Eating too much sodium is the largest contributor to high blood pressure, also known as hypertension, in the United States. Elevated blood pressure significantly increases your risk of heart disease and stroke. According to the ADA, approximately 71 percent of adults with diabetes have hypertension.

Decreasing sodium intake helps lower blood pressure, which in turn lowers your risk of heart attack and stroke. The Dietary Guidelines for Americans recommend that everyone should decrease their sodium intake to 2,300 mg per day or less. However, if you have high blood pressure or diabetes, if you are 51 years old or older or African American, or if you have chronic kidney disease, you should limit your sodium intake to 1,500 mg per day. That's pretty tough to do! However, you can start by checking food labels like the following for their sodium content.

The % daily value for sodium is based on a 2,400-mg amount for the day. If you're trying to decrease sodium, look at the mg amount to compare to your target sodium intake of 1,500 or 2,300 mg per day. If two products are similar, put the higher-sodium product back on the shelf.

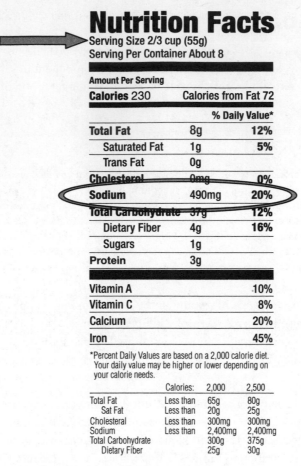

Nutrition Facts

Serving Size 2/3 cup (55g)
Serving Per Container About 8

Amount Per Serving		
Calories 230	Calories from Fat 72	
		% Daily Value*
Total Fat	8g	12%
Saturated Fat	1g	5%
Trans Fat	0g	
Cholesterol	0mg	0%
Sodium	490mg	20%
Total Carbohydrate	37g	12%
Dietary Fiber	4g	16%
Sugars	1g	
Protein	3g	
Vitamin A		10%
Vitamin C		8%
Calcium		20%
Iron		45%

*Percent Daily Values are based on a 2,000 calorie diet. Your daily value may be higher or lower depending on your calorie needs.

	Calories:	2,000	2,500
Total Fat	Less than	65g	80g
Sat Fat	Less than	20g	25g
Cholesteral	Less than	300mg	300mg
Sodium	Less than	2,400mg	2,400mg
Total Carbohydrate		300g	375g
Dietary Fiber		25g	30g

Now let's take a look at some different ways you can limit your sodium intake.

Throw Out the Salt Shaker; It's Already in There

As you know, you can reduce sodium by not adding salt to your food. However, there is still a significant amount of sodium already in food. Other sources of sodium, besides salt, that can be found in foods include the following:

- Sodium benzoate
- Sodium bicarbonate (baking soda)
- Sodium caseinate
- Sodium sulfite, sodium bisulfite, or sodium metabisulfate
- Monosodium glutamate (MSG)
- Sodium citrate

These ingredients have various functions that keep shelf-stable foods the way you expect them to be, with high quality and consistency.

> **DIABETES DECODED**
>
> Salt substitutes and low-sodium versions of prepared foods are usually made from potassium chloride. If you're following a low-potassium diet for your kidneys, you will probably need to limit these foods.

So how can you avoid or limit these sources of sodium? The following are a few tips:

- **Eat out less often.** Restaurant meals can rapidly add up to your entire recommended sodium for the day or more—sometimes much more. In fact, approximately 25 percent of sodium consumed is from restaurant meals. Eating out less keeps you away from sodium-heavy foods. When you do eat out, you can request that salt not be added to your food and ask for sauces on the side that you can then use sparingly.

- **Cook more with whole foods.** The CDC states that Americans get 65 percent of sodium from items purchased in the grocery store; in other words, it's already in the food before preparation and any further seasoning. Therefore, to avoid the high sodium content of processed ingredients, try to purchase fresh ingredients as much as possible.

- **Use salt-free options for seasoning and flavor.** You can use spices, herbs, and lemon juice to get the taste and flavor you desire—no salt shaker required.

Hidden Sodium: Top Salty Surprises

According to the CDC, Americans consume an average of 3,300 mg of sodium daily. The following 10 types of foods contain more than 40 percent of sodium eaten in the United States:

- Breads and rolls
- Lunch meats and cured meats, such as packaged ham, turkey, bacon, salami, canned meats, sardines, and Spam
- Pizza
- Fresh and processed poultry
- Soups
- Deli sandwiches and fast-food burgers
- Cheese

- Pasta dishes

- Meatloaf and other mixed-meat dishes with tomato sauce

- Snacks like pretzels, chips, and popcorn

These foods are not all necessarily high in sodium individually, but the number of servings you eat can make a food a higher source of sodium. For instance, if you have two slices of whole-wheat toast for breakfast and another two slices of whole-wheat bread for a sandwich at lunch, the amount of sodium you consume adds up. Different brands may also vary significantly in sodium content. Some brands contain about 135 mg sodium per slice, while others have a whopping 410 mg per slice. Depending which brand you choose, you could go over your recommended sodium intake for the whole day with just four slices of bread!

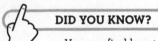 **DID YOU KNOW?**

You can find heart-healthy, lower-sodium recipes from the AHA at heart.org/healthyrecipes or from the ADA at diabetes.org/MyFoodAdvisor.

So when trying to limit your sodium intake, watch out for these foods in particular and take a few more seconds to check the label for sodium content to better limit how much you consume.

The Least You Need to Know

- Saturated fat and trans fat are bad for your heart and raise blood cholesterol.

- Monounsaturated and polyunsaturated fats—particularly omega-3 fatty acids—are heart healthy. The majority of your fat intake should come from these fats.

- Most people eat too much sodium, which can raise blood pressure. Cutting back on sodium may help decrease your risk of heart disease and protect your kidneys from damage.

CHAPTER 15

Low- and No-Calorie Sweeteners

While it sounds great to think that you might be able to eat foods like pie or chocolate with no effect on your blood sugar, it's not really possible. However, terms like *sugar free* or *no sugar added* on labels can add to the confusion of so-called "diabetic" or "dietetic" foods. And depending on the food, the sugar-free version may not be any better for diabetes control than the original version as long as you still keep track of your carbohydrate intake.

In this chapter, we discuss the differences between low-calorie (sugar alcohol) sweeteners and no-calorie (artificial) sweeteners. We also discuss how to decide between choosing a sugar-free food and when the original product might be the right option.

In This Chapter

- Low-calorie and no-calorie sweeteners
- Sugar substitutes in cooking and baking
- Deciding between full-sugar and sugar-free foods

Low-Calorie Sweeteners

Sweeteners that aren't considered no-calorie sweeteners but still contain fewer calories than sugar can be referred to as low-calorie or reduced-calorie sweeteners, the most common of which is sugar alcohol. Low-calorie sweeteners are often combined with no-calorie sweeteners to increase the sweet taste. Foods that are made with low-calorie sweeteners may be helpful in diabetes meal planning because they tend to be a bit lower in calories and may have less carbohydrates than the original version (read labels to be sure).

Sugar Alcohols

Once you start looking, you'll see that sugar alcohols are frequently used in sugar-free foods to reduce calories and lessen blood glucose response. Despite the name, these sweeteners aren't sugar and they aren't alcohol. Sugar alcohols, also known as polyols or sugar replacers, are carbohydrates that have a chemical structure partly similar to sugar and partly similar to alcohol. Sugar alcohols are absorbed more slowly than regular table sugar and aren't completely absorbed in your body. Because of this, they don't have as many calories as regular table sugar. Unlike table sugar or sucrose, which contains 4 calories per gram sugar alcohols can range from as little as .02 calories per gram to 3 calories per gram.

Sugar alcohols commonly used in the United States are the following:

- Erythritol
- Isomalt
- Hydrogenated starch hydrolysates
- Lactitol
- Maltitol
- Maltitol syrup
- Mannitol
- Sorbitol
- Xylitol

You may see one or a combination of these low-calorie sweeteners listed in the ingredients of a sugar-free or no-sugar-added food. Like all food additives, the FDA regulates the use of sugar alcohols. Guidelines are established for safety, labeling information, and nutrient claims (more on food labels in Chapter 13).

DID YOU KNOW?

Sugar alcohols are used in food products in the same volume as sugar. For example, 1 cup of a sugar alcohol would replace 1 cup of sugar. While maltitol and xylitol are about the same sweetness as table sugar, the others are actually a bit less sweet, meaning the product won't be as sweet.

Some of the products you might find sugar alcohols in are chewing gum, breath mints, ice cream, candy, cookies, muffins, and other desserts. You'll also see them in toothpaste, mouthwash, and medicines such as cough drops and throat lozenges. A big plus to sugar alcohols is that they don't cause tooth decay like sugar can. For example, xylitol—often used in sugar-free chewing gum and breath mints—may actually prevent new dental cavities from forming on your teeth.

Sugar Alcohol Side Effects

If you've ever eaten too much sugar-free candy, you probably already know about the unpleasant side effects of sugar alcohols. Because they are only partially digested, the remaining undigested portion is broken down by bacteria in the colon, potentially causing gas, bloating, and diarrhea. In fact, foods made with sorbitol and mannitol carry an FDA-required warning statement to this effect: "Excess consumption may have a laxative effect." This statement appears on labels of sorbitol-containing foods that could contribute to a daily intake of 50 g or more and mannitol-containing foods that can contribute to a daily intake of 20 g or more. Some people are more sensitive to the effects of sugar alcohols than others; while some have few if any symptoms, others might have an upset stomach after eating just a couple pieces of sugar-free candy.

Another side effect of eating sugar-free foods with low-calorie sweetener is overconsumption. Even though sugar-free foods may be used to help you control your calorie intake, the idea that these foods are better for people with diabetes may actually cause you to eat more. For example, if someone offered you sugar-free chocolates, would you take more than if they were regular chocolate because you think they will have less effect on your blood glucose? Somehow the "sugar-free" implies that it's okay to eat it without an adverse effect on your blood sugar. However, if you do eat more of the sugar-free food than the regular food, it defeats the purpose by causing you to eat more calories and more carbohydrates. This can lead to high blood sugar and an upset stomach from eating too much of the sugar-free version!

DIABETES DECODED

It's always an option to choose to enjoy the regular food but eat less. For instance, one Hershey's Kiss candy has about 22 calories and approximately 3 g of carbohydrates, so you wouldn't really see any effect on your blood glucose from eating that. Just remember that portions make a difference!

No-Calorie Sweeteners

No-calorie sweeteners—also referred to as noncaloric sweeteners, non-nutritive sweeteners, artificial sweeteners, sugar substitutes, sugar replacers, or high-intensity sweeteners—are food ingredients added to foods or beverages that provide sweetness with an insignificant amount of calories. Because they are so intensely sweet—100 to 20,000 times sweeter than sugar—only tiny amounts are needed to sweeten foods.

One of the benefits of no-calorie sweeteners is that they don't raise your blood glucose. No-calorie sweeteners may also help you with weight control when they are used in place of sweeteners with calories. If they're just added to foods you normally eat, however, there's no real benefit.

The no-calorie sweeteners currently on the market in the United States are acesulfame potassium (Ace-K), advantame, aspartame, Luo Han Guo fruit (monk fruit) extracts, neotame, saccharin, highly purified stevia, and sucralose. The FDA sets an *acceptable daily intake (ADI)* level to ensure safety of these sweeteners. The following takes you through the different attributes of each type of no-calorie sweetener, including its ADI.

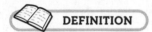 **DEFINITION**

Acceptable daily intake (ADI) is a safety standard set by the FDA for no-calorie sweeteners. The ADI amount includes a 100-fold safety factor; it is 100 times less than the actual amount of a no-calorie sweetener that can be safely consumed on a daily basis over a lifetime, without risk or "no adverse effect."

No-Calorie Sweetener ADI

Sweetener	Sweetness in Comparison to Sugar	Brand Names	Number of Sweetener Packets Equal to the ADI
Acesulfame potassium (Ace-K)	200 times	Sweet One Sunett	165
Advantame	20,000 times		4,000
Aspartame	200 times	NutraSweet Equal Sugar Twin	97
Luo Han Guo fruit (monk fruit) extracts	100 to 250 times	Monk Fruit In the Raw PureLo	No determination

Sweetener	Sweetness in Comparison to Sugar	Brand Names	Number of Sweetener Packets Equal to the ADI
Neotame	7,000 to 13,000 times	Newtame	200
Saccharin	200 to 700 times	Sweet Twin Sweet'N Low Necta Sweet	250
Stevia rebaudiana (reb A), highly purified	200 to 400 times	Truvia Pure Via Enliten	29
Sucralose	600 times	Splenda	165

Data source: Food and Drug Administration

The FDA requires that scientists must determine, typically through multiple research studies, that a no-calorie sweetener meets safety standards prior to its use in the U.S. food supply. There must be "reasonable certainty of no harm." If the FDA decides a no-calorie sweetener poses health risks to consumers, they don't allow its use.

The most commonly used no-calorie sweeteners are Ace-K, aspartame, stevia (reb A), and sucralose. Let's take a closer look at these no-calorie sweeteners so you'll better understand them.

Acesulfame Potassium (Ace-K)

Acesulfame potassium (Ace-K) is approved for use in about 100 different countries worldwide and is available in about 5,000 products. Approximately 100 studies have verified the safety of Ace-K. Ace-K is a stable molecule that holds up well to high heat and can extend the shelf life of products when it's blended with less heat stable sweeteners. It is not metabolized by the body; after it's eaten, it's absorbed but not broken down, so it's excreted unchanged.

You'll see Ace-K included in many reduced-calorie or sugar-free desserts, chewing gum, beverages, gelatin, candy, pudding, light yogurt, and snack foods. It is often blended with sucralose or aspartame because it enhances sweetness and helps prevent the aftertaste from these sweeteners. Even though it has potassium in the name, it doesn't actually contribute to dietary potassium intake.

Some organizations recommend avoiding Ace-K due to potential cancer risk. However, the National Cancer Institute states "The results of these studies [safety studies on Ace-K and other no-calorie sweeteners] showed no evidence that these sweeteners cause cancer or pose any other threat to human health."

Aspartame

Aspartame is one of the most widely tested ingredients in the U.S. food supply and is used in over 90 countries around the globe. You can also find aspartame in the blue packet as a "table-top sweetener" at many restaurants. When it comes to food, aspartame is included in a number of sugar-free desserts, yogurt, pudding, noncarbonated diet drinks (which makes up approximately 70 percent of aspartame consumption), and many other products.

DIABETES DECODED

If you'd rather avoid no-calorie sweeteners and sugar alcohols or just one particular sweetener, that works. You just have to look at the ingredient list to see if they're included in a product. If the ingredient you're trying to avoid is in the list, put that one back on the shelf and choose another.

While over 200 scientific studies verify the safety of aspartame, much controversy still surrounds it. The primary safety concern is about the breakdown of aspartame into two amino acids—phenylalanine and aspartic acid and methanol. This happens so quickly that aspartame doesn't enter into the bloodstream as aspartame, but rather as these components. While it's true that methanol can be toxic in large amounts, the quantity available from the metabolism of aspartame is much less than in many foods. For instance, the American Cancer Society shares the following information about aspartame on their website:

> "[D]rinking a liter of diet soda would lead to consumption of 55 milligrams (mg) of methanol, as compared to as much as 680 mg of methanol from a liter of fruit juice."

That means fruit juice naturally contains over 12 times the methanol as the aspartame-sweetened beverage.

Another concern raised regarding aspartame is the production of formaldehyde during the breakdown of methanol. In a discussion about aspartame, the Academy of Nutrition and Dietetics points out in their Evidence Analysis Library that formaldehyde is produced in your body daily in amounts "thousands of times greater than you would ever get from aspartame." Your body actually needs formaldehyde to help produce other vital compounds. So even though hearing the words *methanol* and *formaldehyde* sound scary, they are actually present in your body whether you choose to eat aspartame or not.

As far as the phenylalanine created by the breakdown of aspartame, only people with phenylketonuria (also known as PKU) need to restrict their intake of this amino acid, though this applies to any source of phenylalanine—not just aspartame.

Stevia (Reb A)

Stevia rebaudioside A (or reb A) is a no-calorie sweetener commonly used in the United States that is derived from the stevia plant. Sweeteners derived from the stevia plant are approved for use in over 80 countries. On food labels, you may see stevia reb A listed as stevia leaf extract, rebaudioside A, or reb A. Because it is derived from a plant, manufacturers list it as a "natural ingredient." Many consider it a healthier alternative to other no-calorie sweeteners. However, the highly processed form used to sweeten foods doesn't even resemble the original plant.

DIABETES DECODED

Many beverages like regular soda, sweet tea, lemonade, and fruit drinks can have more carbohydrates than your entire meal. For example, a large fountain drink-size soda contains about 300 calories and 85 g of carbohydrates. Even a small fountain soda has about 40 g of carbohydrates—that's still about 10 teaspoons of sugar! So, choosing a diet drink to avoid adding any calories or carbs makes sense. If you don't want to consume diet drinks, choose water instead.

Stevia reb A is increasingly becoming available in a number of sugar-free products, including diet sodas, snack foods, candy, yogurt, and more. When in tabletop sweetener form, stevia reb A is typically in the green packet.

There is some confusion about the use and safety of stevia depending on what you are referring to as stevia. In 1991, when the FDA was first approached to approve stevia, instead of achieving approval, it was banned for use in the United States due to concerns it caused cancer. However, a later study disproved the original study, and whole-leaf stevia or "crude stevia extracts" were allowed to be sold as dietary supplements in the United States; this remains the only approved use today. However, reb A is a highly purified form of stevia that is allowed for use as a food ingredient.

Sucralose

Sucralose is derived from sugar but is not recognized in the body as a carbohydrate. Because of that, it's poorly absorbed, so most of the sucralose you eat is not metabolized and is excreted in the urine. Sucralose is approved for use in 80 countries worldwide. It's included in more than 4,000 products, and over 100 studies have verified the safety of sucralose.

Sucralose is used in sugar-free candy, meat products, milk products, baked desserts, diet sodas, noncarbonated diet drinks, yogurt, pudding, canned fruit, and more. It can be found in the yellow packet as a tabletop sweetener.

One organization, the Center for Science in the Public Interest (CSPI), downgraded their organization's safety rating of sucralose based on an unpublished study in mice. This study demonstrated the increased risk of leukemia in mice fed sucralose over their entire lifespan. However, many researchers have dismissed this study due to flaws in design. CSPI still takes the position "people are better off drinking diet rather than regular sugar-sweetened sodas" because health results from regularly drinking sugary sodas—such as obesity, heart disease, and type 2 diabetes—are probably greater.

No-Calorie Sweetener Baking Substitutions

No-calorie sweeteners can be used in cooking and baking to reduce the amount of carbohydrates in your recipe. Stevia (reb A), sucralose, and Ace-K are all heat stable and can be used in high-temperature cooking and baking. While aspartame won't hurt you if you use it under high heat or in baked goods, it isn't heat stable and leaves a bitter taste. However, it may be added at the end of the cooking time in some recipes.

Using a no-calorie sweetener in place of a cup of sugar in a recipe saves 200 g of carbohydrates and almost 800 calories. However, make sure to double-check the label of the product you're using to see how much you need to replace the amount of sugar in your recipe.

The following are some tips for successful sugar substitutions:

- No-calorie sweeteners can usually replace the full amount of sugar in recipes for fruit pie fillings, sauces, glazes, and beverages.

- In baking, substituting no-calorie sweeteners for sugar can affect texture, browning, flavor, and cooking time. Using a sugar and no-calorie sweetener baking blend (like Splenda Sugar Blend or Truvia Baking Blend) will yield a more successful product and still decrease the sugar content by 50 percent.

- For yeast breads, activate yeast with 2 teaspoons of sugar before using the no-calorie sweetener. Brushing an egg wash (1 egg plus 1 tablespoon water) on top of the bread prior to baking will help maintain browning.

- When using a no-calorie sweetener in a cookie recipe, you may need to flatten cookies with a fork before baking because the cookies won't spread like the full-sugar kind. Sprinkling cinnamon on top helps develop the browning color.

Remember, if you weren't eating desserts before and now you're adding these lower-sugar versions, you're still eating extra calories. Therefore, only use no-calorie sweeteners to save you carbs and calories in a recipe that's replacing a full-sugar version.

DID YOU KNOW?

Misinformation about no-calorie sweeteners is plentiful on the internet. Remember, if there's no credible source listed, it is likely not to be true. If the person posting the information states that nothing can ever convince them that the sweetener (or fill in the blank) could be safe, that indicates they're not interested in facts or evidence. Use the resource list in Appendix B to find credible sources for more information.

Choosing Between Full-Sugar and Sugar-Free Foods

Figuring out whether to choose a sugar-free food or the usual food is sometimes not an easy task. However, the FDA has guidelines for manufacturers to follow that will help you gather the information you need to make the best decision.

Reiterating what you learned earlier in this part about labeling, the following are the FDA guidelines in regard to how sugar is categorized:

- **Sugar free:** The food contains less than .5 g sugar per serving. Sugar is not included as an ingredient.

- **Reduced sugar or less sugar:** The food is at least 25 percent lower in sugar than the appropriate reference food (for example, reduced-sugar ketchup). If the manufacturer reduces it by more than 25 percent, they can state it on the package (for example, 30% less sugar).

- **No added sugars or without added sugars:** Sugar or sugar-containing ingredients weren't added during the processing of the food. The reference food would have to include added sugars to be able to use this claim. If it's not lower in calories, the label must state "not a low-calorie [food]" or "not a reduced-calorie [food]."

- **Unsweetened and no added sweeteners:** These must be factual statements (for example, 100 percent fruit juice with no added sweeteners or unsweetened applesauce).

Because sugar free doesn't equal calorie free, it may also help to understand the label definition for calorie claims:

- **Calorie free:** The food contains less than 5 calories per serving.

- **Low calorie:** The food contains 40 calories or less per serving.

- **Reduced calorie:** The food must have at least 25 percent fewer calories than the appropriate reference food.

Sugar-free foods may still contain a significant amount of carbohydrates. So after you see the claim on the label, you need to look a bit further to the Nutrition Facts section to see how it fits into your meal plan.

DIABETES DECODED

If there is just one type of sugar alcohol used as an ingredient in a food, you will see it listed in the Nutrition Facts section of the label, as well as in the ingredient list (for example, xylitol). However, if the food contains more than one type of sugar alcohol, you will see the words *sugar alcohol* listed in the Nutrition Facts label, with each type listed separately in the ingredient list.

For example, here's a comparison of two ice cream Nutrition Facts labels—one for light vanilla ice cream and the other for no-sugar-added vanilla light ice cream:

Vanilla Light Ice Cream
Nutrition Facts
Serving Size 1/2 cup (63g)
Serving Per Container About 4

Amount Per Serving

Calories 100	Calories from Fat 32
	% Daily Value*
Total Fat 3.5g	**5%**
Saturated Fat 2g	**10%**
Trans Fat 0g	
Cholesterol 20g	**7%**
Sodium 45mg	**2%**
Total Carbohydrate 15g	**5%**
Dietary Fiber 0g	**0%**
Sugars 11g	
Protein 3g	

Vitamin A	3%
Vitamin C	0%
Calcium	6%
Iron	0%

*Percent Daily Values are based on a 2,000 calorie diet. Your daily value may be higher or lower depending on your calorie needs.

	Calories:	2,000	2,500
Total Fat	Less than	65g	80g
Sat Fat	Less than	20g	25g
Cholesterol	Less than	300mg	300mg
Sodium	Less than	2,400mg	2,400mg
Total Carbohydrate		300g	375g
Dietary Fiber		25g	30g

Vanilla Light, No Sugar Added Ice Cream
Nutrition Facts
Serving Size 1/2 cup (63g)
Serving Per Container About 4

Amount Per Serving

Calories 90	Calories from Fat 27
	% Daily Value*
Total Fat 3g	**5%**
Saturated Fat 2g	**10%**
Trans Fat 0g	
Cholesterol 10mg	**3%**
Sodium 70mg	**3%**
Total Carbohydrate 13g	**4%**
Dietary Fiber 2g	**8%**
Sugars 4g	
Sugar Alchohol 5g	
Protein 3g	

Vitamin A	6%
Vitamin C	0%
Calcium	7%
Iron	0%

*Percent Daily Values are based on a 2,000 calorie diet. Your daily value may be higher or lower depending on your calorie needs.

	Calories:	2,000	2,500
Total Fat	Less than	65g	80g
Sat Fat	Less than	20g	25g
Cholesterol	Less than	300mg	300mg
Sodium	Less than	2,400mg	2,400mg
Total Carbohydrate		300g	375g
Dietary Fiber		25g	30g

Serving size: Check to make sure you are making a true comparison and that the serving sizes are the same. In this case, both types of ice cream have a $^1/_2$-cup serving size.

Calories: Note that the calories for the ice creams are not that different—the no-sugar-added version has just 10 calories less than the light ice cream.

Fat: Both types of ice cream are very similar in fat: one has 3 g and one has 3.5 g. They have the same amount of saturated fat content, and neither one has any trans fat.

Total carbohydrate: The no-sugar-added version has just 2 g less of total carbohydrate compared to the light ice cream. It also has 2 g of dietary fiber, whereas the light ice cream doesn't have any. Dietary fiber is included in no-sugar-added ice cream to make it seem more like the original version. Fiber is generally added to maintain a similar texture, bulk, stabilization, and "mouthfeel" (the way the ice cream feels in your mouth) when sugar is not added. Continuing on, you'll see how the sugars add up to affect the total carbohydrate content. While the light ice cream has 11 g of sugar, the no-sugar-added version has 4 g of sugar and 5 g of sugar alcohol. Sugar alcohols and no-calorie sweeteners are both used to replace part of the sugar in the no-sugar-added ice cream.

 DIABETES DECODED

You may have heard that sugar alcohols don't "count" and that they can be subtracted from the total carbohydrate. Because they still have about half the effect on your blood glucose as regular carbohydrates, half of the sugar alcohol content could be subtracted only if the total is greater than 5 g. If it's less than 5 g, there is really no significant difference for most people with type 2 diabetes. And if your goal is to lower both calories and carbohydrate intake and to help control your weight, it's best not to subtract any of the sugar alcohols from the total—especially if it means you would take a bigger serving to make up for the lower amount of carbohydrates!

In this case, both types of ice cream could fit into your meal plan, particularly if you stick with the serving size of $^1/_2$ cup. As you can see, the sugar-free or no-sugar-added product doesn't always make much of a difference. Read labels and compare to find out!

The Least You Need to Know

- Sugar alcohol is used in sugar-free foods to reduce calories and lessen blood glucose response.

- Because no-calorie sweeteners can be 100 to 20,000 times sweeter than sugar, only tiny amounts are needed to sweeten foods.

- With a few adjustments, no-calorie sweeteners can be used in cooking and baking to reduce the carbohydrate content of recipes.

- When trying to decide whether to go with a sugar-free or full-sugar treat, compare your choices by checking the Nutrition Facts label for serving size, calories, fat, and total carbohydrate.

Other Healthy Eating Tips

As you learned previously, protein—specifically lean protein—is an essential component of your diet. Drinking enough water and eating enough fiber and whole grains are also key to getting on track with your eating. But why should you, and how can you, include more?

In this chapter, we delve into a bit more detail on protein, including how to find alternatives to high-fat meats and how to prepare lean meats. We also discuss how drinking more water may help with weight loss and blood glucose control. We then get into the benefits of fiber and whole grains, as well as the many high-fiber and whole-grain foods available to you.

In This Chapter

- Selecting and preparing lean meats
- Why drinking water is important
- Increasing fiber and whole grains

Going Lean with Protein

If you've already decided to choose more lean meats and other low-fat protein foods, that's great! However, if you're not sure where to begin after being told "don't eat red meat" by your doctor, for example, you're not alone. And choosing a good lean meat is only half the battle. After all, you can only have skinless, boneless chicken breast cooked on the grill so many times until you're bored with it. By covering lean-meat alternatives to high-fat (or "sometimes") meats and teaching you how to prepare lean meats, we hope we get you moving in the right direction for your diabetes health.

 DID YOU KNOW?

The AHA has a voluntary certification program to indicate certain foods are heart healthy and fit into an overall healthy eating pattern. Qualifying foods display the Heart-Check mark. There are eight extra-lean types of beef cuts that meet the AHA's requirements: extra-lean ground beef (96 percent lean, 4 percent fat); bottom round steak (USDA Select grade); sirloin tip steak (USDA Select grade); top sirloin petite roast, boneless (USDA Select grade); top sirloin strips (USDA Select grade); top sirloin filet (USDA Select grade); top sirloin kabob (USDA Select grade); and top sirloin steak, boneless, center cut (USDA Select grade).

"Sometimes" Meats

Sizzling sausage patties, crisp strips of bacon, a nice juicy rib-eye steak—are these on your list of favorite foods? If you're a meat lover and don't want to cut out meat completely, you may be wondering what to do. First off, not all red meat is the same as far as its effect on your heart health. Some beef is quite lean and can be included in your meal plan more frequently. However, higher-fat meats, such as pork products, should be eaten less often. We'll refer to these higher-fat meats as "sometimes" meats—meaning you should only eat them some of the time and not regularly include them in your day-to-day eating.

The following table lists "sometimes" meats with suggested leaner substitutions. Keep in mind that many of these substitutions are not automatically lower in sodium. However, there are lower-fat, lower-sodium options available that still provide great flavor. Read labels to find out which are the best.

Lean-Meat Alternatives to "Sometimes" Meats

"Sometimes" Meat	Lean-Meat Alternative
Bacon	Canadian bacon, ham, or extra-lean turkey bacon
Sausage	Reduced-fat turkey or chicken sausage
Ground beef	Ground beef that is at least 95 percent fat free or ground turkey breast that is at least 95 percent fat free
Cold cuts, such as bologna, salami, pepperoni, olive loaf, and summer sausage	Lunch meat that is at least 95 percent fat free—such as roast beef, turkey, chicken, or ham
Hot dogs	Low-fat, 97 percent fat-free, or fat-free hot dogs with sodium under 450 mg
Beef, such as chuck, brisket, prime rib, rib-eye, porterhouse, and ribs	Eye of round, top sirloin, sirloin tip, top round, bottom round, or sirloin filet
Pork, such as spare ribs, baby-back ribs, pork shoulder, and pork belly	Top loin roast, tenderloin, center loin chop, or loin chop
Dark-meat chicken and turkey with skin	White-meat chicken or turkey without skin
Breaded, fried fish	Baked, broiled, poached, or grilled fish

 DIABETES DECODED

Just because some foods, such as low-fat hot dogs, are better than the regular ones doesn't mean they're health food. While making the lower-fat choice is a great place to start on your stepwise changes, including meats less often in general and not making them the focus of your meal would be the next step. We also recommend choosing fish as a protein source more frequently. As an alternative, selecting plant-based protein in place of animal protein is good for your heart and your diabetes control. See the vegetarian meal-planning section in Chapter 17 for more information.

Preparing Lean Meats

If you've ever chewed on a flavorless, dry chicken breast or a tough cut of beef, you know how important it is to cook meat properly! With lean meats—particularly lean beef and white-meat chicken or turkey without the skin—preparing them in the right way can make them taste great, even without adding fat.

Parboiling: This is a way of partially cooking chicken to shorten the dry-heat (baking or grilling) cooking time. It ensures the chicken gets cooked through while keeping it moist. This can also be a good timesaver if you like to keep individual chicken breast portions in the freezer.

The following are the steps for parboiling:

1. Place the chicken breasts in a saucepan that can easily hold the pieces you're cooking.

2. Add water until it covers the chicken.

3. Bring the water to a boil over medium heat, and continue to boil for about seven minutes.

4. Reduce heat and allow to simmer for about three minutes; the chicken shouldn't be cooked through. Remove the chicken from the water.

5. Brush the chicken with barbeque sauce, teriyaki sauce, or marinade, or use a dry rub to season. Finish the chicken on the grill or in the oven until cooked to a minimum of 165°F.

Boiling: This is similar to parboiling, except in this case you're fully cooking the chicken by allowing the water to boil longer. This works well for chicken you're cooking to use in recipes or to freeze to use later. If you'd like more flavor added to the chicken, you can cook it in a reduced-sodium broth instead of water, add seasoning (like garlic, herbs, lemon or lime juice), or include vegetables (such as onion, celery, and carrots).

Fully cooked boiled chicken pieces can be used in stir-fry or fajitas, tacos, and more, and diced chicken can be added to a homemade soup. For a tasty salad, you can cut up the chicken and add it to salad greens with some sliced apples or pears, a few dried cranberries, some walnuts, and a light balsamic vinaigrette dressing.

The following are the time frames you should follow when boiling chicken:

- For skinless, boneless chicken breast halves, boil 15 to 20 minutes.

- For a whole skinless, boneless chicken breast, boil about 10 minutes.

Marinating: To keep lean beef, pork, game meats, or lamb tender, you can marinate them prior to cooking. Marinades are seasoned liquid mixtures that add flavor to meat, fish, or poultry. A small amount of olive oil or canola oil can be added to a marinade so seasonings (such as ginger, chili powder, or anything that sounds good to you) adhere to the meat and the meat browns during cooking. (Add oil sparingly if you need to keep your calories in control.)

Here are a few tips for successful marinades:

- Use approximately $^1/_4$ to $^1/_2$ cup of marinade for each 1 to 2 pounds of meat.

- To keep the meat at a safe temperature, marinate it in the refrigerator. Any leftover marinade should be thrown out.

- When it comes to marinating times, seafood should be marinated about 30 minutes to 1 hour, boneless chicken breast approximately 2 hours, pork about 4 hours, lamb from 4 to 8 hours, and beef up to 24 hours.

- A glass dish, plastic container, or heavy-duty plastic bag works best for holding the marinating liquid. It's not a good idea to use a metal pan because it can give a metallic taste to the meat.

- To help tenderize less tender meat cuts, the marinade needs to contain an acidic ingredient. You can use a citrus juice like fresh-squeezed lemon or lime juice, tomato juice, low-sodium vegetable juice, salsa, vinegar, buttermilk, or yogurt, to name a few.

- You can toss seasoning in the marinade to taste—for instance, pepper, garlic, onion, and herbs.

Lean meats don't have to be dry and tasteless. Get creative and try new flavors in marinades. Don't be afraid to experiment. Some of the best recipes are created that way!

 DID YOU KNOW?

One way to tenderize larger pieces of meat such as boneless, skinless cuts of turkey or chicken, pork, beef, or game meats (as well as shorten the cooking time) is to pound it out. Place the meat between two pieces of plastic wrap and pound with the smooth side of a meat mallet until uniformly thin. If you don't have a mallet, you can use the bottom of a heavy pan or rolling pin.

Drinking Enough Water

A high percentage of your body weight is water. Your age, gender, and body composition all affect your body water percentage. It ranges from around 50 to 80 percent, but on average it's 60 percent. Babies have the highest percent of body weight from water—close to 80 percent. If you have a larger muscle mass, you also have higher body water content. Meanwhile, an older adult or overweight person may have closer to 50 percent body weight from water. No matter your content percentage, the water in your body is located in three main areas: inside your cells, in the space between your cells, and in your blood. Almost two thirds of your total body water is inside the cells.

Water is important to your health because all the cells, tissue, and organs in your body contain water. That's why it is so critical to get enough water every day.

Water has several functions in your body, including the following:

- Regulates your body temperature

- Lubricates and cushions your joints

- Helps protect your spinal cord and brain

- Dissolves substances so cells can process nutrients

- Helps deliver oxygen throughout your body

- Gets rid of waste, mainly through urine

When you're healthy, it's easier to get the right amount of fluid by drinking water and other beverages and even eating different foods. If you're sick or your blood glucose is high, however, it may be difficult to get enough water, and staying hydrated becomes even more important.

Hydration and Blood Sugar

How many glasses of water do you drink each day? You've probably heard that you should drink eight 8-ounce glasses of water a day. Have you ever wondered if that's really true? While it's a good rule of thumb and easy to remember, the amount of fluid you actually need varies depending on the circumstances.

DIABETES DECODED

Many foods provide water. In fact, about 20 percent of your water needs are met through foods you eat. Foods like cucumbers, celery, melons, tomatoes, carrots, berries, and oranges all have high water content. Sounds like yet another reason to eat your fruits and veggies!

You need to take in water (other no-calorie beverages count, too) to replace the amount your body loses during daily functions. Water is lost when you go to the bathroom and when you sweat. Even when you breathe, you exhale out small amounts of water. Situations that require additional water above your daily requirements are when it's hot outside, during exercise, and when you have a fever, diarrhea, or vomiting.

Another time you need to increase your water intake is when you're blood glucose is elevated. High blood glucose causes you to lose more water through excessive urination, so you need to replace that loss to prevent getting dehydrated. Dehydration can make hyperglycemia worse because not enough fluid is available for the kidneys to produce more urine to clear out glucose. While just drinking a glass of water doesn't lower your blood glucose, if you stay hydrated when you're sick and other times you have high blood glucose, you can prevent more serious problems from happening. (See Chapter 6 for more information on lowering your blood glucose.)

How Water Can Help You Lose Weight

When you're healthy, thirst usually cues you to drink fluids to maintain adequate hydration. If you're good about drinking fluids throughout the day and your urine is light yellow or colorless, you're probably adequately hydrated (though older adults need to make a conscious effort to drink more water because sense of thirst diminishes with age).

If you're not drinking enough fluid on a regular basis, you tend to feel tired. You might also feel hungry, especially if your blood glucose is high, because your body thinks you need more food for energy. It may sound odd, but it is actually easy for your body to get mixed signals about feeling hungry and feeling thirsty. You may tend to eat as a response to this cue, particularly if you think the food will make you feel less tired, when all you really need is something to drink. Replacing the fluid your body needs to function can help you feel less tired and potentially curb your hunger cravings.

Of course, the drinks you choose make a difference. On average, adults (and kids) take in an extra 400 calories a day in beverages, which can add up quickly. But by choosing water and other calorie-free drinks instead of high-calorie, sugary drinks, you can be on your way to losing weight.

The following are a few suggestions to increase your water intake:

- Carry a water bottle with you when you leave your house, and keep a water bottle in your car when running errands or at your desk at work. This gives you easy access to water and is a good visual reminder.

- Choose water instead of other drinks when you eat out. Not only can you reduce your calorie intake, you'll save money, too.

- If you don't like the taste of plain water, add a bit of flavor with lemon, lime, orange, or cucumber slices. As an alternative, you can purchase a no-calorie flavoring to add to your water. They are available in a variety of different flavors and come in liquid or powder.

> **DIABETES DECODED**
>
> You may have heard that caffeinated beverages don't count toward your daily fluid total because caffeine is a diuretic. Actually, caffeine has little to no effect on increasing fluid loss. That doesn't mean it's okay to swap out all of your water with coffee; there are still negative health consequences to consuming too much caffeine. But you can certainly count your morning cup of coffee or tea as part of your fluid intake for the day.

While drinking water throughout the day is helpful, drinking water right before meals may also help you eat less. In one study, drinking two glasses of water before meals helped participants ages 55 to 75 years old lose more weight than those who didn't drink the water before meals. They felt full more quickly and ate fewer calories at the meal. It's important to point out that all participants, drinking extra water or not, followed a low-calorie meal plan. Is drinking water before meals the miracle solution to weight loss? No, but it's certainly something that's easy to try, and it won't cost you anything!

Getting More Fiber in Your Diet

Fiber is only found in plant foods. It's the part of the plant that gives it structure. While your body doesn't digest or absorb fiber, it plays an important role in digestion. In fact, you've probably been told a time or two that you need to eat more fiber to "keep you regular." So how can fiber help you, and how much should you eat?

Types of Fiber and Benefits

There are two kinds of dietary fiber in foods and both are beneficial to your health: insoluble and soluble fiber.

Insoluble fiber is the type more people are familiar with. Sometimes referred to as *roughage,* it's called *insoluble* because it doesn't dissolve in water. Insoluble fiber is most helpful with digestion. This type of fiber adds bulk to your stool, increasing the movement of food waste through your intestines. Adding bulk to your stool makes it easier to pass, preventing constipation and keeping you regular. Good sources of insoluble fiber include bran, whole grains, nuts, potatoes, broccoli, popcorn, and other plant foods.

Soluble fiber dissolves in water to form a gel-like substance, which slows down digestion and helps you feel full longer. Plus, by delaying digestion, it slows the absorption of carbohydrates and helps prevent a quick rise in blood glucose after a meal. Soluble fiber is also especially helpful in lowering LDL (bad) cholesterol and may reduce blood pressure. You can find soluble fiber in oats, apples, beans, barley, oranges, carrots, and other healthful foods.

Adequate intake of both these types of fiber helps decrease the risk of developing heart disease, diseases of the colon, and obesity.

How to Increase Your Fiber Intake

It's estimated that more than 90 percent of children and adults in the United States don't eat enough fiber. So how much fiber should you be eating? The recommended amount is 14 g of fiber per 1,000 calories per day. That means most adults should be eating somewhere between 25 and 30 g of fiber per day. You can find out how much fiber is in one serving of a food by checking out the dietary fiber information listed directly under total carbohydrate on the Nutrition Facts panel.

Fiber is included in fruits, vegetables, and whole grains. These are all great foods for a diabetes meal plan. However, just like with other sources of carbohydrates, they can raise your blood glucose and contribute to excess calories if you just add them in to what you're eating now. So to give yourself the best health benefits, replace less healthful carbs with more fiber-rich foods.

Here are some tips for adding more fiber (and whole grains, which we'll discuss next) to your meal plan:

- Look for breakfast cereals with at least 5 g of dietary fiber.

- Choose plain air popped or light microwave popcorn for a healthy whole-grain and high-fiber treat.

- Choose fruit for a snack, such as berries, pears, or apples.

- Sprinkle wheat bran in soups, yogurt, hot cereal, muffins, and casseroles.

- Have a small handful of nuts and seeds for a snack.

- Cook with beans and legumes more often; you can use them in soups, main dishes, or in side dishes added to brown rice or whole-wheat pasta.

- Add veggies to your sandwich. Don't stop with just lettuce and tomato; add on some cucumber slices, red peppers, spinach, or shredded carrots.

- Cook more stir-fry dishes, adding any vegetable combination you like, and serve with brown rice or another whole grain.

- Include salads with your meals more often.

- Choose crackers with a whole grain—wheat, rye, or rice—listed as the first ingredient.

 FOR YOUR SAFETY

When starting to increase your fiber intake, do it gradually over a few weeks' time. If you increase your fiber suddenly, you may experience bloating, gas, and discomfort. And if you don't increase your fluid when you increase your fiber intake, you may worsen constipation instead of making it better. Be particularly careful with high-fiber snack bars; if you eat more than one, it may be too much.

Consuming Whole Grains Wholeheartedly

Grain foods include any that are made from wheat, rice, oats, corn, as well as other cereal grains. A number of foods are made from grains, but that doesn't make them whole-grain products or necessarily good for your health. For instance, many products are made from refined grains, which means that during processing, the bran and the germ are stripped away from the whole grain. This process also removes nutrients like vitamins and iron from the grain. This is usually turned into flour that is bleached white (peroxides and chlorine can be used in this process) and some B vitamins and iron are added back in. This leaves you with bleached, enriched flour. You may see "wheat" bread made from unbleached, enriched flour, which is basically white flour that's not bleached white.

DIABETES DECODED

If you'd like to begin using whole-grain flours, start experimenting by substituting $\frac{1}{4}$ to $\frac{1}{2}$ of the flour in your recipe with a whole-grain version.

On the other hand, whole-grain products that are made from whole-grain flour include the entire grain—the bran, endosperm, and germ. While some products are made from refined grains with a few whole grains added in, this doesn't provide the same health benefits as true whole-grain food. To make sure the product you're choosing is a good source of whole grains, look for a whole grain as the first ingredient on the list. Whole-wheat flour, rolled oats, whole oats, and whole rye are examples of whole grains you might find on an ingredient list.

Benefits of Whole Grain

It's recommended to make half your grains whole, with at least three servings a day. The more whole grains are studied, the more the health benefits from whole grains are validated. The following are some benefits you can gain from eating more whole grains:

- Whole grains can help lower the risk of developing heart disease, obesity, and type 2 diabetes.

- A recent study even found that eating whole grains decreases the risk of dying from a heart attack.

- The fiber in whole grains also helps you feel full, so you may eat less.

- Whole grains are good sources of the B vitamins thiamin, riboflavin, and niacin. B vitamins are important for nerve function, metabolism, digestive health, skin, and eye health.

- Minerals in whole grains include iron, magnesium, and selenium. Iron helps form hemoglobin, which carries oxygen in your blood. Magnesium helps with energy production and nerve transmission, while selenium is an antioxidant that helps your immune system function.

Whole Grains to Try

Grocery stores are increasingly stocking their shelves with a variety of different grains. The following are three whole grains that are good to get in your diet.

Quinoa: There are a surprising number of products made from the popular grain quinoa (pronounced *keen-wha*). You can find this grain in everything from crackers to beverages. Quinoa provides a complete protein, which is rare in plant foods. It's also high in potassium and gluten free, which is a bonus if you need to follow a gluten-free diet. When ready to use, rinse quinoa before cooking to remove any bitterness. Quinoa cooks in just 15 minutes. When it's done, the germ sticks out—it looks like a little white curl or tail. Quinoa can be added to soups and salads, mixed with vegetables or beans, or served just by itself with your favorite seasoning as a side dish.

Bulgur: This is precooked wheat that has been broken into pieces. The FDA requires that products labeled bulgur are whole bulgur (whole wheat). Bulgur has a mild, nutty taste and is easy to prepare. You can prepare bulgur in several different ways, such as microwaving, cooking, boiling, or soaking. To boil, add boiling water or broth to bulgur (about $1^3/_4$ to $2^1/_2$ cups of liquid per 1 cup of bulgur) and cook it in a covered pot for about 20 to 25 minutes with the amount of liquid and cooking time depending on the type (fine, medium, or coarse). It can be used many ways, including in salads, side dishes, pilaf (with or without rice), or hot cereal.

Barley: A shining star when it comes to grains is barley. Beta-glucan fiber from barley, which has been the focus of a number of research studies, is a soluble fiber that has been shown to help lower the blood glucose response after a meal. It may be useful in diabetes prevention and management and has been shown to lower blood pressure and LDL (bad) cholesterol.

So how do you find barley and what do you do to use it? The most common variety of barley you'll find used in the United States is pearl barley. This is barley that has had its tough outer layer removed, and with it much of the outer bran. While whole-grain pearl barley, with its outer hull still on, is the most nutritious, it requires a long cooking time due to the tough hull. So if you'd like to use the whole-grain type of pearl barley, it's a good choice to add to bean soup, because the beans and the whole-grain pearl barley both have similar cooking times. Look for hulless, dehulled, or hulled barley for shorter cooking times. Even hulled pearl barley, not in its whole-grain form, has a number of health benefits, more so than other refined grains. Barley flour may be used in recipes to increase the fiber content; $^1/_2$ cup of barley flour has 7 g of fiber, or more than triple the amount of white flour. Barley can also be used in salads, side dishes, main dishes, muffins, pancakes, and more.

The Least You Need to Know

- Cooking lean meats with the right techniques can keep them tender and flavorful.
- Drinking enough water can help you control hunger symptoms and is beneficial for weight management.
- Increasing fiber from fruits, vegetables, and whole grains in your meal plan can have significant health benefits, including better digestion.
- Regularly choosing whole grains lowers your risk of developing heart disease and obesity. Whole grains may also decrease the risk of dying from a heart attack.

Diabetes Meal Planning

There seems to be an endless number of diet plans for diabetes management and weight loss. However, starting and stopping diets to achieve short-term success doesn't help your health in the long run. In this part, you learn the difference between dieting and planning your meals to meet your diabetes and weight-loss goals.

We start by explaining the glycemic index and discussing four popular eating patterns that have proven benefits when it comes to blood glucose control. You'll find that one size doesn't fit all when it comes to choosing your individualized plan. This part also shares successful strategies and nondiet approaches for weight management, as well as quick, diabetes-friendly meal and snack ideas, to help you achieve and maintain a healthy weight. We then wrap it all up with how to assess your efforts and make corrections as needed to get the payoffs you're looking for.

Choosing the Right Meal-Planning Option

There is no one "diabetic diet." Multiple options are available for successful diabetes meal planning. You may end up choosing ideas from more than one type of meal-planning option, which can work well, too. And by including foods you enjoy and want to continue eating in your meal plan, you will help yourself stay on track long term.

In this chapter, we review available evidence and meal-planning options to help you decide the best way for you to manage your blood glucose and to meet your additional health goals.

In This Chapter

- Diabetes meal planning that works
- Counting carbs
- The glycemic index of foods
- Plate method, low-carb, Mediterranean, and vegetarian meal plans

Making Your Diabetes Meal Plan Work for You

When you have diabetes, meal planning is about controlling blood glucose, blood lipids, and blood pressure and promoting overall health and wellness. But if you're not able to follow a meal plan because it's too restrictive or requires you to eat foods you don't like, you won't meet your goals. The most important factor is that the meal plan works for you and takes into account your preferences.

For instance, if you are a meat-and-potatoes person, you're not likely to choose a vegetarian meal plan; however, you might decide you can include more vegetables in your everyday eating. Likewise, if you're a vegetarian, you're not likely to choose a low-carb meal-planning option. The good news is you don't have to. Successful diabetes management can be achieved in a variety of different ways.

Nutrition recommendations from the ADA apply scientific evidence that help focus your diabetes meal-planning strategies. The following is a summary of key messages from the current guidelines, to give you a basic outline for your meal plan. We've touched on a number of these topics throughout the book, but they're all in one place here!

- Portion control is important for all foods, not just carbohydrate foods.

- Don't skip meals; this can lead to hypoglycemia and overeating later in the day.

- Eat moderate amounts of carbohydrates for meals (and snacks, if you like to include them).

- Choose fewer processed foods (especially those high in fat and sodium), solid fats, and sugary foods, and avoid sweetened beverages.

- Include lean meat and meat alternatives; high-nutrient, high-fiber foods like whole grains, fruits, and vegetables; and liquid fats.

- Limit your sodium intake to 2,300 mg per day (other guidelines recommend 1,500 mg per day).

- Vitamin and mineral supplements, herbal products, or cinnamon aren't recommended to manage diabetes due to lack of evidence.

- Limit alcohol to moderate drinking (up to one drink a day for women or up to two drinks a day for men).

- If you use mealtime insulin, learn carbohydrate counting or another meal-planning approach to determine carbohydrate intake. Match your mealtime insulin to the amount of carbohydrate in the meal.

- If you use a premixed or fixed insulin plan, your meals need to be eaten at about the same time each day and contain about the same amount of carbohydrates.

These nutrition strategies can be applied to any of the meal plans discussed in this chapter. Keep these in mind while you read through the options. Some of these strategies are "built in" to the meal planning, but not all of the strategies are included in each one. Your personal food choices still make a difference for your diabetes management and any additional health and fitness goals.

Counting Carbs

Because the amount of carbohydrates eaten (more than the type of carbohydrates) has the biggest effect on your blood glucose, controlling how many carbohydrates you eat helps keep your blood glucose from going too high. Carbohydrate counting, otherwise known as carb counting, is a technique that's frequently used for diabetes meal planning. It's flexible because any source of carbohydrate can be included. By combining carb counting with blood glucose monitoring, you can quickly learn how various foods affect your blood glucose.

Remember, any food with starch or sugar in it contains carbohydrate. Those foods include the following:

- Starchy foods (such as cereal, bread, potatoes, rice, and pasta)
- Sweets (such as cakes, pies, cookies, and candy)
- Fruit
- Milk
- Yogurt

Nonstarchy vegetables only include a small amount of carbohydrates, so unless you're eating large portions at a time, they don't have to be counted.

You Have a Choice—a Carb Choice, That Is!

Carbohydrates can be counted in g—which you can find listed next to "Total Carbohydrate" on the Nutrition Facts food label—or in choices. A carbohydrate or carb choice is a portion of a carbohydrate food that's equal to 15 g of carbohydrate. Carb choices are used on food lists where similar foods are grouped together; these come in handy for foods without labels (such as fresh fruit).

 DIABETES DECODED

Many popular cell phone apps offer food trackers that include carbohydrate content of foods. Apps like Calorie Counter & Diet Tracker by My Fitness Pal, Carb Master, and Daily Carb Premium are just a few of the apps available. Many are free or low cost and can be good tools to keep you on track.

Though sweets and snack foods aren't the best choices nutritionally, they don't have more of an effect on your blood glucose than other sources of carbohydrates do. Of course, the portion size might be different though. For instance, if a food is highly concentrated in sweetness, it will have a smaller portion for 15 g of carbohydrate. So whereas you can eat $1^1/_4$ cups of cubed watermelon, you only get one 2-inch square piece of cake without frosting for the same amount of carbohydrates. Sometimes it's worth it though!

Still unsure of how carb choices work? Take a look at the following table to see examples of food portions equal to 15 g of carbohydrate, or 1 carb choice.

Common Carbohydrate Foods in Portions Equal to 15 g of Carbohydrate

Breads and Grains	Starchy Vegetables and Beans	Fruit	Milk and Yogurt	Sweets and Other Carbs
1 oz. bread (1 slice bread, 1 6-in. tortilla, $^1/_2$ English muffin, or 1 dinner roll)	$^1/_2$ cup cooked peas, corn, mashed potatoes, sweet potatoes, or parsnips	$1^1/_4$ cups whole strawberries or cubed watermelon	1 cup nonfat, low-fat, or whole milk	1 TB. regular pancake syrup, sugar, or honey
$^1/_2$ cup oatmeal, grits, or other cooked cereal	1 cup cooked winter squash (acorn or butternut)	1 approximately 4-oz. pear	6 oz. light yogurt (made with no-calorie sweetener) or plain yogurt	2 2-in. cookies
$^1/_3$ cup cooked pasta, rice, or quinoa	$^1/_2$ cup cooked beans or legumes (pinto, kidney, or black beans)	$^1/_2$ cup canned fruit packed in its own juice	1 cup plain soy milk	1 2-in. square piece of cake, without frosting
1 (4-in.-wide) pancake	$^1/_3$ cup ripe cooked plantain	2 TB. raisins		$^1/_2$ cup light ice cream
$^3/_4$ cup ready-to-eat cereal (serving sizes vary; check label)	3-oz. baked potato, any type	1 cup raspberries		1 frozen fruit juice bar
3 cups air-popped popcorn	1 cup cooked mixed vegetables (corn, peas, and carrots)	$^3/_4$ cup blackberries		15 potato chips

On average, most men should choose about 4 to 5 carbohydrate choices per meal, or 60 to 75 g of carbohydrate. Most women should choose about 3 to 4 carbohydrate choices per meal, or 45 to 60 g of carbohydrate. If you like to include snacks, women should aim for 15 g of carbohydrate, while men should aim for 15 to 30 g of carbohydrate. However, it's okay if your snacks include little to no carbs.

Carb-Counting Sample Menu

Now that you know what carb choices are, let's take a look at a sample menu for a one-day meal plan. The menu contains 45 to 60 g of carbohydrate (3 to 4 carb choices) for each meal, and up to 15 g of carbohydrate for each snack.

 DIABETES DECODED

Make sure to read labels for carbohydrate content. When eating out and at home, it can be easy to forget to count carbs from foods like breading on chicken, bread crumbs added to meatballs, and sauces. Plus, meals eaten out may be much higher in carbs than when you eat at home. If you can't figure out why your blood glucose is high after a meal, these forgotten carbs might be the explanation.

One-Day Sample Menu for Carb-Counting Meal Planning

Meal	Menu	Carbohydrate Grams	Carbohydrate Choices
Breakfast	**Breakfast Sandwich:** 1 whole-grain English muffin 1 oz. 2% milk 1 scrambled egg 1 oz. Canadian bacon	30	2
	1 cup nonfat milk	12	1
	1 small orange	15	1
Snack	1 TB. peanut butter and 2 medium celery stalks	6	0

continues

One-Day Sample Menu for Carb-Counting Meal Planning   (continued)

Meal	Menu	Carbohydrate Grams	Carbohydrate Choices
Lunch	$^2/_3$ cup cooked brown rice; 1 cup stir-fry vegetables; and 3 oz. skinless, boneless chicken breast	30	2
	2 tsp. teriyaki sauce	Free	Free
	$^3/_4$ cup blackberries	15	1
	6 oz. plain yogurt	12	1
Snack	3 cups air-popped popcorn sprinkled with 1 TB. grated parmesan cheese	15	1
Dinner	4 oz. grilled sirloin steak, 6 oz. baked potato, and 1 TB. light margarine (trans fat free)	30	2
	Spinach Salad: $1^1/_2$ cups spinach 1 cup sliced strawberries 1 oz. feta cheese crumbles 2 TB. light salad dressing	15	1

Portions shown here may not be the right amount for you. Check with your medical provider or RD/RDN to individualize.

I'm sure you're wondering what foods marked as "free" mean. Free foods are any foods containing less than 20 calories and 5 g or less of carbohydrate. Free foods can be added to your meal plan without counting them because they have little to no effect on your blood glucose. The following are considered free foods; any that have serving sizes listed with them should be limited to no more than three servings a day:

Coffee

Tea

Diet soda

No-calorie sweeteners

Gelatin

Sugar-free gum

Jam or jelly (light or no sugar added), 2 tsp.

Jam or jelly (regular), 1 tsp.

Sugar substitutes (low-calorie sweeteners)

Cream cheese (fat free), 1 TB.

Creamers (nondairy, liquid), 1 TB.

Creamers (nondairy, powdered), 2 tsp.

Salad dressing (fat free or low fat), 1 TB.

Salad dressing (fat-free Italian), 2 TB.

Barbecue sauce, 2 TB.

Catsup (ketchup), 1 TB.

Mustard

Salsa, $^1/_4$ cup

Taco sauce, 1 TB.

Using the Glycemic Index

The glycemic index (GI) ranks foods on a scale of 0 to 100 based on the rise in blood glucose after eating. The faster and greater the rise in the blood glucose, the higher the score is for that food. Foods like white bread, pretzels, and instant oatmeal have a high GI because they are quickly digested, causing blood glucose to rise more rapidly. On the other hand, foods like rolled oats, pears, and oranges have a low GI because they are more slowly digested, resulting in a more gradual increase in blood glucose. The following table shows you the GI of some common foods.

Glycemic Index of Common Foods

Low-GI Foods (55 or Less)	Medium-GI Foods (56-69)	High-GI Foods (70 or More)
Oatmeal (rolled or steel-cut)	Bananas	White bread or bagels
Pasta, barley, and bulgar	Cantaloupe	Corn flakes, instant oatmeal, or cream of wheat
Corn, peas, legumes, and lentils	Grapes	Quick-cooking white rice
Oranges, peaches, and pears	100% whole-wheat bread (some brands)	Pretzels and saltine crackers

continues

Glycemic Index of Common Foods   (continued)

Low-GI Foods (55 or Less)	Medium-GI Foods (56-69)	High-GI Foods (70 or More)
Carrots and most nonstarchy vegetables	Quick-cooking oats	Baked potatoes
Snickers candy bar	Brown, wild, or basmati rice and couscous	Watermelon

Not all low-GI foods are healthy choices and many high-GI foods are, so you still need to pay attention to the nutritional value of foods when following the GI. It is also difficult to know which foods are high and which foods are low unless you have a list to refer to. For instance, not all pastas are the same; spaghetti has a higher GI than fettuccini. Other factors affecting the GI of foods are the length of cooking time, if the food is eaten alone or with a mixed meal, if fat is added to the food, how ripe a fruit is, which brand is eaten, and the variety of a grain (for example, short-grain versus long-grain rice). With all the variables affecting the GI of foods, it can take a lot of effort to fully implement this technique to track your foods.

Also, total carbohydrate still counts as far as blood glucose management goes. If you only pay attention to the GI of a food, your carbohydrate intake can vary widely. Knowing the glycemic load of a food will help you better predict the effect on your blood glucose because it factors in the amount of carbohydrates along with the GI.

$$\text{Glycemic load} = (\text{glycemic index of the food} \times \text{g of carbohydrate in the food}) \div 100$$

Here's an example using a small apple. An apple has a GI of 40 and the carbohydrate content is 15 g.

$$\text{Glycemic load} = 40 \times 15 \div 100 = 6$$

Foods that have a low glycemic load are from 1 to 10; a moderate glycemic load is from 11 to 19; and a high glycemic load is 20 or higher. The lower the glycemic load, the less effect there is on your blood glucose. So you can see that a small apple has a low glycemic load. In order to use this method, you need to have a list of GI for foods you eat, as well as know the carbohydrate content of the foods.

There's one additional option to start incorporating the GI into your meal plan if you're currently counting carbs. To do this, you would continue with carb counting but just start including low-GI foods in place of high-GI foods. Try switching foods for equal amounts of carbohydrates, such as 1 cup of instant oatmeal for 1 cup of cooked steel-cut or rolled oats for breakfast in the morning. Test your blood glucose before and two hours after each of the meals to see if your blood glucose is lower after the low-GI food meal. If you start seeing improved blood glucose control from including the low-GI foods, you could then continue adding more low-GI foods into your daily routine.

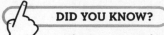
The Plate Method Meal Plan

You may remember the plate method from our discussion in Chapter 12. To get started, you first need to take a look at what your plate usually looks like now. If you recall, your plate should be 9 inches; if the plate you're using is a lot bigger than that, it's time to begin using a smaller plate. This will help you eat less right away and is particularly helpful if you're trying to lose weight. (If you are younger and more active and don't need to lose weight, you'll need to use a bigger plate than what's discussed here.)

Beyond plate size, the key to using the plate method for meal planning is balancing out the calories to more healthful food choices. By making half of your plate fruit and vegetables, you automatically have less room for starchy foods and oversized protein food choices, as you can see in the following image.

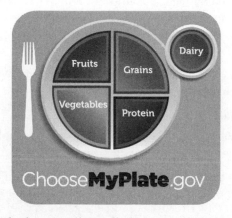

By following the plate method, you will usually have two to three carb choices, which equals 30 to 45 g of carbohydrate. However, if you stick with the recommended plate portions, you don't have to do any counting. Remember, the portions on your plate are directly in line with your carbohydrate intake; if the portions get out of hand, so will your carbohydrates.

What If You Don't Like Vegetables?

If the idea of having half a plate with mostly vegetables on it makes you cringe, making yourself eat a large serving of salad or steamed vegetables as a side dish isn't the way to go. However, because veggies are packed with valuable nutrients and few calories, you should work on including more of them in your meal plan.

Understanding why you don't eat them now will help you figure out ways to eat them more often. For instance, think about the reason you're not eating vegetables. Is it the taste (such as bitterness)? Is it the mushy texture? Are they too much of a hassle to prepare? Or were you forced as a kid to sit at the table until they were gone? Whatever the reason, there are solutions. The following are some suggestions to increase your vegetable intake based on why you might not be eating them now:

Taste (or lack of it): Try vegetable dishes with spices and seasonings that you like on other foods. If you like the flavors, they may taste good on veggies, too. Using small amounts of a light ranch or blue cheese dressing as a dip is one way. Better yet, use a light vinaigrette dressing made with olive oil. A small amount of healthy oil (like olive or canola oil), a pinch of salt and pepper, or a drizzle of light balsamic vinaigrette dressing are additional options that can give veggies a tasty flavor. Or you can just chop up, dice, or blend veggies in with some of your favorite foods to incorporate them with a taste you already like; suggested veggies for this are onions, mushrooms, zucchini, and carrots.

Preparation time: If the main reason you don't eat vegetables is the prep time, you may want to purchase the washed and ready-to-eat varieties. Plus, it's less expensive to get the prewashed versions if you usually end up throwing out all your produce because it goes bad. Another way is to add veggies to what you're already preparing. Spaghetti, chili, and soup work well to sneak in extra veggies. For instance, you can throw in a handful of frozen broccoli, carrots, or green beans when you're heating up soup for a quick veggie boost without having to prepare an additional side dish. Frozen vegetables are also a great time-saver. You can take them out of the freezer and use them as needed; a splash of water and a few minutes in the microwave is all you need to prepare them.

Texture: If you don't like the texture of cooked veggies, eat them raw. Don't settle for just carrots and celery; you can cut up cucumbers, tomatoes, zucchini, cauliflower, broccoli, or radishes to get a nice, crunchy variety. Avoid overcooking vegetables so they don't turn to mush; steaming or stir-frying is a better option than boiling to maintain texture. Grilling vegetables also creates a nice texture; try large pieces of zucchini, eggplant, asparagus spears, or portobello mushrooms and cook them directly on the grill. Or if you like vegetable juice, you can drink your veggies. Just look for the lower-sodium juices; tomato and regular V-8 juice are high in sodium.

DIABETES DECODED

Be careful not to overcook cruciferous vegetables such as broccoli, cauliflower, cabbage, and Brussels sprouts. They give off a sulfur-smelling odor when overdone.

Pick one or two of the suggestions you think will work from any of these areas and try them out.

Plate Method Sample Menu

It can be easy to get stuck for meal ideas that fit the plate method if you think each type of food needs to stay in the respective places on the plate. However, one-dish meals, sandwiches, soups, and mixed dishes work well with the plate method, too. The following one-day menu shows you a variety of ways you can put together a meal using the plate method.

One-Day Sample Menu for Plate Method Meal Planning

Breakfast	1 cup cooked oatmeal
	1 TB. raisins
	$^1/_2$ cup nonfat milk
	1 hardboiled egg
Snack	1 small apple
Lunch	1 cup vegetable soup
	$^1/_2$ roast beef sandwich on whole-wheat bread with lettuce, tomato, and 2 tsp. light mayonnaise
	2 small mandarin oranges
Snack	6 oz. light yogurt
Dinner	**Chicken Tacos:**
	3 oz. boiled, shredded chicken
	2 (6-in.) corn tortillas
	2 TB. salsa (mix into chicken)
	Toppings:
	1 TB 2% milk cheddar cheese
	Lettuce and tomato
	$^1/_4$ cup peach or mango salsa
	1 TB. light sour cream
	Salad:
	$^1/_2$ cup shredded cabbage
	$^1/_4$ cup diced peppers (green, yellow, or red)
	$^1/_4$ cup shredded carrots
	2 TB. light salad dressing

Portions shown here may not be the right amount for you. Check with your medical provider or RD/RDN to individualize.

When planning your plate, remember to choose a variety of whole grains, fruits, vegetables, lean protein sources, and nonfat or low-fat dairy foods. Think about the balance of your plate and what, if anything, is missing. Does it look like the plate in the picture? If your plate is out of balance, consider which foods need to be added. You can never go wrong by adding more non-starchy vegetables!

The Low-Carb Diet Meal Plan

The words *low-carb diet* mean different things to different people. There are various schools of thought as to how many carbohydrates should be consumed daily. The IOM sets the recommendations that determine the Daily Values used on the Nutrition Facts food label. According to the IOM, the daily value for carbohydrates is 300 g, which is based on a 2,000-calorie diet. Though this recommendation is made for general health, the IOM also has a recommended minimum intake of 130 g of carbohydrate per day. This minimum number is based on the needs of the *central nervous system* for glucose.

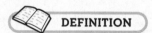 **DEFINITION**

> The **central nervous system** is made up of the brain and spinal cord. It's the part of the nervous system that coordinates the activity of the entire nervous system, which includes the peripheral nervous system and central nervous system. The central nervous system needs glucose, generated from carbohydrates, to use for fuel.

Low-carbohydrate diets are generally much lower than 130 g of carbohydrate. When carbohydrate intake drops too low, ketones form to be used for fuel in place of glucose. However, the ketones produced in response to a low-carbohydrate diet aren't as dangerous as when someone experiences DKA (see Chapter 2). Low-carbohydrate diets have been demonstrated to promote weight loss and improve cholesterol, triglyceride, and blood glucose levels.

How Low Can You Go?

While low-carbohydrate diets do show the benefits we've mentioned, almost any diet leading to weight loss would likely show improvement in those same measures. The concerns about very-low-carbohydrate diets (around 50 g of carbohydrate per day or less) are about what happens with long-term use.

The central nervous system needs glucose, generated from carbohydrates, to use for fuel. While the central nervous system and brain can adapt to using ketones for fuel, restricting carbohydrates to very low levels to promote ketone production can cause too much protein intake and potentially saturated fat intake, depending on food choices. The high protein content of the diet may increase the risk of osteoporosis and kidney stones. Some studies have also shown a decrease in thyroid function with very-low-carbohydrate diets as well. If you're not careful to get enough fiber, digestive problems can also occur.

Plus, extreme carbohydrate restriction doesn't make sense nutritionally. For example, possibly the most well-known low-carb diet is the Atkins Diet. Per the Atkins website, the first phase of the Atkins Diet starts with 20 to 40 g of "net carbs" per day, depending on which plan you choose. Net carbs are calculated by subtracting fiber and sugar alcohols from the total carbs. Additional carbs are gradually added until eventually the target net carbs reach 80 to 100 g per day. The first phase can last six months or more, depending on your weight loss goals. That means you could restrict carbs to around 30 to 35 g of carbohydrate per day, depending on how many high-fiber foods you choose. However, with all the positive health benefits from whole grains, fruits, and vegetables, why would you want to restrict carbs that much? You'll definitely be missing out on some key nutrients.

Low-Carb Sample Menu Including Whole Foods

While reducing carbohydrate intake can be an effective strategy to manage diabetes and promote weight loss, a more moderate carbohydrate restriction can also provide benefits while maintaining a balance of nutrients. Most people eat significantly more carbohydrates than 130 g a day, so cutting back to that level should help reduce calories and improve blood glucose control. If you're already limiting carbohydrates and you'd like to go lower, this amount may be reasonable for you. By choosing whole foods including fresh vegetables, fruit, whole grains, and healthy fats, this meal plan could also be an option that will meet your nutritional needs long term. A sample menu is provided here that contains approximately 130 g of carbohydrate for the whole day, so you can see if it looks reasonable.

 DIABETES DECODED

It's a good idea for you to track how many carbohydrates you eat each day before deciding your target carbohydrate level when trying the low-carbohydrate meal-planning approach.

One-Day Sample Menu for Low-Carb Meal Planning

Breakfast	2 eggs cooked with 1 tsp. olive oil
	2 cups spinach cooked with 2 tsp. olive oil
	1 cup cubed mango with 2 TB. chopped walnuts

continues

One-Day Sample Menu for Low-Carb Meal Planning (continued)

Snack	4 medium stalks celery 2 TB. cashew butter
Lunch	**Chinese Chicken Salad:** 3 oz. grilled chicken breast 1 cup romaine lettuce 1 cup Napa cabbage 1 TB. slivered almonds 1 peeled clementine orange (in segments) 3 TB. sesame ginger dressing $^1/_3$ cup cooked brown rice, cooled (add to salad)
Snack	6 oz. plain Greek yogurt mixed with $^1/_2$ cup raspberries
Dinner	5 oz. grilled salmon 1 cup kale and 1 cup mixed salad greens, mixed with 1 TB. olive oil and 2 tsp. balsamic vinegar 1 yellow squash cut into thin slices and grilled with 1 TB. olive oil $^1/_2$ cup cooked quinoa

Portions shown here may not be the right amount for you. Check with your medical provider or RD/RDN to individualize.

The Mediterranean Diet Meal Plan

The Mediterranean diet got its name because the foods included reflect the style of eating in countries lining the shores of the Mediterranean Sea. The traditional Mediterranean diet is well recognized for reducing the risk of heart disease. This style of eating also reduces the risk of death from cancer and helps prevent type 2 diabetes. However, if you already have diabetes, there are benefits, too, as this eating plan has been shown to slow the progression of type 2 diabetes.

According to Oldways, a nonprofit group that promotes the Mediterranean diet, there are eight key steps to this eating style:

- Eat lots of vegetables.

- Change the way you think about meat.

- Enjoy some dairy products.

- Eat seafood twice a week.

- Cook a vegetarian meal one night a week.

- Use good fats.

- Switch to whole grains.

- For dessert, eat fresh fruit.

 DIABETES DECODED

Make sure to stock up your pantry with Mediterranean-friendly ingredients. Keep raw vegetables and fresh fruit on hand for snacks and use extra-virgin olive oil for the best, fresh olive flavor.

Replacing Meat as the Main Focus

With this meal plan, meat such as pork, chicken, and steak take a backseat to other main-dish options. Fish in particular is a mainstay of the Mediterranean and often the first thing you associate with this meal plan. Fresh- or water-packed tuna, trout, mackerel, salmon, and herring are some of the traditional fish options that are high in omega-3 fatty acids. Other fish popular in the Mediterranean include tilapia, flounder, yellowtail, and sea bass. Seafood such as clams, crab, lobster, mussels, octopus, oysters, shrimp, and squid are also great choices. But forget about that Captain's platter—fish and shellfish aren't usually breaded and fried in Mediterranean countries! Instead, this meal-planning style includes fish that is grilled, baked, poached, or broiled.

Beyond fish, there are other dishes you can create that fit into the plan where meat is not the main focus. For example, you can try main dishes made with beans, whole grains, and vegetables. Grains to experiment with for a Mediterranean flair include the following:

- Barley

- Buckwheat

- Bulgur

- Couscous

- Farro

- Millet

- Oats

- Polenta

- Rice

- Whole-grain breads and pastas

But what about those times when you truly want meat? When you decide to eat meat, choose smaller portions such as small strips of steak with grilled vegetables. You can use Mediterranean herbs and spices to liven up your food and reduce salt at the same time. Commonly used herbs and spices are anise, basil, cloves, cumin, fennel, garlic, marjoram, mint, oregano, parsley, pepper, rosemary, sage, tarragon, and thyme.

The Rest of the Mediterranean

Vegetables are another mainstay of a Mediterranean eating plan. They're used fresh with a drizzle of olive oil, in salads with herbs and garlic, or grilled and mixed with whole grains. You can enjoy the tastes of the Mediterranean with tons of veggies, including the following:

- Artichokes
- Arugula
- Beets
- Broccoli
- Brussels sprouts
- Cabbage
- Carrots
- Cucumbers
- Eggplant
- Fennel
- Kale
- Leeks
- Mushrooms
- Onions
- Peas
- Peppers

- Potatoes

- Pumpkin

- Radishes

- Rutabaga

- Spinach

- Sweet potatoes

- Tomato

- Turnips

- Various greens, such as spinach and kale

- Zucchini

When it comes to sweets, this diet encourages saving desserts and sweets for special occasions or celebrations and choosing fresh fruit for a snack or dessert instead. Traditional Mediterranean fruits that can give you sweetness without a lot of calories include apples, apricots, cherries, clementines, dates, figs, grapefruits, grapes, melons, nectarines, oranges, peaches, pears, pomegranates, strawberries, and tangerines.

The Mediterranean style also includes yogurt and cheese, but in smaller portions. In terms of yogurt, choose low-fat and nonfat plain yogurt or Greek yogurt. As for cheeses, traditional options include brie, chevre, feta, manchego, Parmigiano-Reggiano, pecorino, and ricotta.

Healthy fats are also a signature staple of a Mediterranean meal plan. Extra-virgin olive oil, nuts, peanuts, sunflower seeds, olives, and avocados are all things you can consume to gain those healthy fats.

Mediterranean Sample Menu

Traditional Mediterranean meal plans are higher in fat than what's usually recommended for heart health. The key is using healthy fats in place of typical saturated fats—for example, substituting olive oil in place of butter. The following table shows you a one-day sample menu of how you can eat on the Mediterranean diet.

One-Day Sample Menu for Mediterranean Meal Planning

Breakfast	2-egg omelet with sliced green pepper, onion, and mushroom, sautéed in 1 tsp. olive oil 1 medium pear, sliced
Snack	1 cup baby carrots 2 TB. hummus
Lunch	2 oz. water-packed tuna 3 marinated artichoke heart quarters 5 kalamata olives 1 TB. feta cheese crumbles Sliced red onion to taste 2 cups mixed salad greens drizzled with extra-virgin olive oil and balsamic vinegar 1 (6-in.) whole-wheat pita bread
Snack	6 oz. plain Greek yogurt 2 dried apricot halves, diced
Dinner	2 oz. grilled chicken $^2/_3$ cup whole-grain pasta with 1 cup grilled vegetables brushed with olive oil Asparagus, tomato, and zucchini tossed with 1 TB. olive oil and 1 oz. shaved Parmigiano-Reggiano cheese 1 cup cubed watermelon

Portions shown here may not be the right amount for you. Check with your medical provider or RD/RDN to individualize.

The Vegetarian Meal Plan

There are a number of advantages to eating vegetarian when you have diabetes. In fact, studies related to vegan (strict vegetarian) meal plans have demonstrated that even without reducing carbohydrates or calories, blood glucose control improved. Why is that? Because vegan eating patterns are typically much higher in fiber—almost triple the average U.S. intake. This helps slow down digestion and absorption of carbohydrates, decreasing the rise in the blood glucose after a meal.

Have you been thinking of going meatless but don't know where to start? While you may be ready to trade those animal foods in for a vegetarian meal plan, it's usually best not to give up all animal foods at once so the transition is easier. Start by giving up the animal foods you'll miss the least first. It also helps to make a list of vegetarian meals you already prepare and enjoy. You might be surprised at how many there are. Think of meals you make that would work without the meat, and add more beans and veggies to those dishes to slowly make them more vegetarian.

Becoming Vegetarian: You Decide

There are different types of vegetarianism. The most common ones are the following:

- **Lacto-ovo vegetarian:** Eats dairy products and eggs

- **Lacto-vegetarian:** Eats dairy products

- **Ovo-vegetarian:** Eats eggs but not dairy products

- *Vegan:* Doesn't eat dairy, eggs, or any other animal products

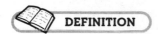 **DEFINITION**

> **Vegans** are vegetarians who don't eat any animal products. They also don't use any products with animal-based ingredients. For example, many vegans avoid honey and don't use products made with wool, silk, or leather.

If you choose to not follow any of these types and continue to include some animal foods, that's fine, too; you get to decide. You can still achieve improved health even if you choose to be a flexitarian (also called *semi-vegetarians*), where you follow a predominantly plant-based diet but occasionally eat small amounts of meat, poultry, or fish.

On the other end of the spectrum, you may choose to avoid all animal products and become vegan for different reasons, including health, ethical and environmental issues, concern for animals, and cost. A vegan meal plan can be less expensive because meats tend to be the highest-costing grocery items. While following a vegan diet can certainly be a healthy option, it might not be if you don't make the right choices. Including a variety of fruits, vegetables, whole grains, leafy greens, nuts, legumes, and seeds becomes even more important to get the nutrients you need. Plus, you still need to cut back on empty calorie foods like sweets and snack foods.

To see which level is right for you, get a few vegetarian cookbooks or check online for recipes and start experimenting with different vegetarian meals. Find recipes that are somewhat familiar and that fit your cooking style to begin with, so you can make a truly informed decision on what works for you.

Tastes Like Chicken—TVP, Tempeh, and Tofu

A simple way to incorporate more vegetarian meals into your diet is to substitute plant-based proteins for the animal protein in your favorite recipes. For example, you can turn a meat dish vegetarian by using meat substitutes such as soy-based hamburger-like crumbles or textured vegetable protein (TVP). These products can also be used in spaghetti, lasagna, chili, soup, and tacos, to name a few. Firm tofu can be used in place of chicken in soups, stir-fry, or curry dishes with brown rice.

Most people are more familiar with tofu, but tempeh is also a soy protein not to be overlooked. Tempeh has a firm texture and a nutlike flavor and is low in sodium. Like tofu, it easily picks up the flavor of marinades or other foods with which it is cooked.

 DIABETES DECODED

> Don't mistake the silken tofu for the firm kind. The silken type has a creamy texture and works better in sauces, smoothies, or dips.

Vegetarian Sample Menu

Even on a vegan diet, you can still use some time-savers when it comes to preparing foods at home. For example, because beans are a staple protein of vegetarian cooking, using canned or frozen can be quicker and easier than their dried counterparts. Also, more grocery stores are starting to offer whole grains such as brown rice and quinoa frozen and prepared without seasoning, too. Even though the price of convenience is higher, it's still less expensive than the cost of eating out. The following is a one-day sample menu that follows a vegetarian meal plan.

One-Day Sample Menu for Vegetarian Meal Planning

Breakfast	$^3/_4$ cup firm tofu, scrambled, with 1 tsp. olive oil and $^1/_2$ cup spinach, sliced mushroom, and onion
	$^1/_2$ cup cubed cantaloupe
	1 slice whole-grain bread
	1 TB. natural peanut butter
	1 cup plain, fat-free, and calcium fortified soy milk
Snack	10 tortilla chips
	2 TB. salsa

Lunch	1 cup bean and barley soup
	2 cups mixed-green salad with shredded carrots, cucumbers, and tomato; add 1 TB. olive oil, 1 tsp. balsamic vinegar, and pepper to taste
	8 Triscuit crackers
Snack	1 oz. almonds
	1 medium orange
Dinner	**Vegan Burger:**
	1 vegan burger patty
	Whole-wheat bun
	Tomato, lettuce, and onion
	Homemade baked "fries" made from 3 oz. potatoes brushed with olive oil and sprinkled with garlic powder and paprika
	1 TB. Heinz Organic Ketchup or similar brand
	1 cup cooked broccoli
	$^3/_4$ cup blueberries

Portions shown here may not be the right amount for you. Check with your medical provider or RD/RDN to individualize.

To find out more about vegetarian and vegan meal planning, check out the following websites:

- **Vegetarian Nutrition Dietetic Practice Group of the Academy of Nutrition and Dietetics:** vegetariannutrition.net

- **Vegetarian Resource Group:** vrg.org

- **Physicians Committee for Responsible Medicine:** pcrm.org

 DIABETES DECODED

If you are struggling with how to plan meals and need assistance with figuring out the best option, request a referral from your medical provider to see a registered dietitian/nutritionist (RD or RDN). It's best to find one who has experience in diabetes management so you get meal-planning advice specific to your needs.

The Least You Need to Know

- There are many different diabetes meal-planning options that can help you reach your goals, such as plate method, low-carb, Mediterranean, and vegetarian.

- Monitoring carbohydrate intake is a key strategy for all diabetes meal-planning strategies.

- When choosing a meal-planning option, keep in mind your preferences and what you're more likely to stick with in the long run. Make sure to include foods you enjoy.

CHAPTER 18

Watching Your Weight

If you're like many people with type 2 diabetes, losing some weight would be beneficial for you to improve your blood glucose and reach your health goals. While you can use any of the meal plans mentioned in Chapter 17 for weight loss, this chapter goes over some helpful considerations specific to weight loss to aid you in tipping the scale in your favor. Even if you don't need to lose weight, you'll find information to help you eat mindfully and ideas for quick, healthy meals and snacks on the go.

In This Chapter

- Not going on a diet
- How mindless eating affects your waistline
- Healthy eating in a hurry

Why "Diets" Don't Work

The cabbage soup diet, the cookie diet, the lemonade diet—if you can think of a name for a potential diet, it has probably existed at one time or another! Diets like these set you up for failure. Just by going *on* a diet, it implies there's a time you'll go *off* the diet. How dedicated can you be to something that's just temporary? Also, you'll see many diets make claims like "lose 30 pounds in 30 days." However, you can tell by the claim that the product manufacturer doesn't have your well-being in mind. Remember, if it sounds too good to be true, it probably is!

That's why time and time again, people don't reach their goals on a diet. By adapting your lifestyle to be more active and choosing more healthful foods, you're committing to your health and wellness, not just losing weight quickly on the next diet. With that approach, you're more likely to stick with it.

> **DID YOU KNOW?**
>
> The National Weight Control Registry is a database of over 10,000 people who have lost weight and kept it off. To continue to keep the weight off, the majority report following a low-fat, low-calorie meal plan with increased activity. In addition, 75 percent eat breakfast every day; 75 percent weigh themselves at least once a week; 62 percent watch less than 10 hours of TV a week; and 90 percent are physically active, averaging one hour of daily exercise.

Making Healthy Eating a Long-Term Goal

If you've already tried going on diets and have not achieved long-term success, you know that diets don't work. While it's easy to get caught up in the hype of the sales pitch and think that it might be different next time, the advertisements, magazine articles, and diet books all promote products or diets that aren't good for your health and lead to failure by design. It's not you that has failed; it's the diet that has failed. Therefore, it might be time to try a nondiet approach to healthy eating. If you throw out the idea that a better diet or a better diet pill will be just around the next bend, you can allow yourself to choose to eat healthfully. You won't be forced to do it because you're on a diet.

Key to this nondiet approach to eating is remembering to give yourself permission to not be perfect. You will choose unhealthy foods. While it will happen from time to time, that doesn't make you a bad person. You won't gain weight by overeating one day. If you're not on a diet, you don't have to feel like you've gone off or "cheated" on the diet. How you eat over time—choosing foods that nourish your body and making an effort to feel better and more energized—is what counts. Eat for your health, not simply a short-term goal!

Having Control Over Your Food

Having diabetes may make you feel even more guilt over the consumption of certain foods because you are aware of how they can negatively affect your blood glucose. But what if, right now, you gave yourself complete and unqualified permission to eat whatever foods you like, in whatever quantities you want? How do you feel? Do you feel in control? If you tell yourself that you shouldn't have a certain food, it can make you feel deprived. You may feel like you want to rebel and eat it anyway. Or it may just lead to cravings for the food until you give in and eat it, even though you know you shouldn't. That usually leads to overeating and guilt.

If you remind yourself that it's your choice whether you eat or don't eat a certain food, it loses its power over you. For example, if a whole plate of warm chocolate brownies is sitting in front of you and you truly believe you can eat as many of them as you want, you won't feel like you have to eat as many. You are in control and you have power over the food; it doesn't have power over you. And if you choose to eat a formerly off-limits food, enjoy it, and don't feel guilty about it! The guilt is what drives you to eat more. It is fine to give yourself permission to let go of the guilt; dealing with diabetes is more than enough!

Mindful Eating—Enjoying Food More While Eating Less

According to the Center for Mindful Eating, *mindfulness* means deliberately paying attention in a nonjudgmental way and being present in the moment. Mindfulness includes awareness of thoughts, emotions, and physical sensations. Eating mindfully includes doing the following:

- Using all of your senses in choosing foods that are satisfying and nourishing to you

- Becoming more aware of physical signs of hunger and fullness, which helps you decide when it's time to start and stop eating

- Acknowledging there is no right or wrong way to eat—rather, there are varying degrees of awareness related to the experience of food

- Directing your attention to eating in the current moment

Eating mindfully means increasing your awareness of the entire eating experience. To eat mindfully, you need to be fully engaged, moment by moment, for each sensation during eating, chewing, tasting, and swallowing.

Are You a Mindless Eater?

Do you feel like you're always in a hurry with meals? Do you tend to eat too fast? Do you routinely eat your dinner on the couch while watching television? Americans not only eat too fast, but also tend to eat while multitasking, often working through lunch or eating in the car while driving. Adults in the United States also spend almost twice as much time watching television than they do eating each day. This type of distracted, mindless eating often leads to eating more. For example, one study examined behavior of people eating popcorn at a movie. Invariably people ate more when they ate the popcorn out of a larger container, even when the popcorn served was intentionally stale. The distraction of watching the movie while having more popcorn available contributed to the moviegoers eating too much (stale) popcorn.

 DIABETES DECODED

Research done at Cornell University indicates people consume up to 500 calories a day mindlessly. Mindless eating not only leads to eating excess calories, it can contribute to elevated blood glucose. By becoming more aware of what you're eating, you can save those calories, enjoy your food more, and get better blood glucose control at the same time.

Another factor in mindless eating is not being in tune with your body's physical sense of hunger and fullness. The mind-body connection plays an intricate role in eating behavior. With true physical hunger, your brain and stomach exchange signals that trigger behavior. You start to feel weak and fatigued, and your stomach rumbles and growls; you then respond by seeking out and eating food. When you eat the food, the hunger signals go away, you feel better, and the same system signals fullness. However, if you ignore the signals of fullness and keep eating, you'll get too full. And if you eat too quickly, you won't feel it until after you eat, leading to you potentially feeling overly full later.

Additionally, your mood and other factors can also cause interference with this signaling process, contributing to eating without hunger. If you tend to eat just because it's time to eat, eat due to boredom, or if you automatically eat all the food on your plate, you need to get more in tune with your feelings of hunger and fullness. By not being able to tell when you're truly hungry or when you're truly full, you'll tend to overeat. On the other hand, you can also overeat if you put off your feelings of hunger and don't respond to them until you're extremely hungry. Once you get to the point of excessive hunger, all good intentions go out the window. Recognizing early signals of hunger helps you trust your body's signals of when and how much to eat, as well as identify when you're truly hungry instead of just having a craving.

How to Eat Mindfully

If you've recognized you're a mindless eater and you'd like to become a more mindful eater, you'll see that a lot has to do with how quickly you eat. Slowing down your eating allows you to be more aware and to enjoy your food more. Here are some tips to slow down your eating:

- **Watch the clock.** Have you ever noticed how quickly you eat a meal? Lengthen the time of your meal to a minimum of 20 minutes.

- **Eat at a table for meals and snacks.** Set the table and make it look attractive so you'll be more likely to stay there for a while.

- **Sit down when you eat.** You need to stay seated at the table in order to focus on your meal; don't get up and walk around while eating.

- **Eliminate distractions.** Don't check emails, watch television, or send texts. Simply think about eating slowly and enjoying your food.

- **Match your pace to a slower eater.** If someone at the table is eating slower, slow down to match her speed.

- **Put down your fork between each bite.** This helps you savor your food and chew your food more thoroughly.

- **Cut the food into smaller pieces.** By having your food in multiple pieces, it seems like you're getting more.

- **Eat with your nondominant hand.** This forces you to eat more slowly.

As you use these tips, try to stay focused throughout your meal. Be aware though that it's human nature for your mind to wander. If you notice your mind drifting off, just refocus and return to the awareness of chewing, tasting, and swallowing. Savor the flavor and the experience!

DIABETES DECODED

By eating more slowly, you will be able to sense when you're getting full. That way, you can stop eating before you become overly full later on. So before you grab a snack or take a second helping, stop and ask yourself if you're eating more due to hunger or some other reason.

Hurried Eating

It happens to everyone. Sometimes you just don't have time for a relaxed sit-down meal. Maybe you're on the road or traveling by air, where you don't have access to your kitchen and pantry. Or maybe you've forgotten to take your lunch to work, and you're standing in front of the vending machine, tempted to just get something from that. Whatever the reason, learning to make the best food choices, in most any circumstance is a good skill to develop.

What's Best to Grab and Go?

With the fast pace of life, it's hard to keep up with having the right foods available at the right time. In many cases, you might default to buying a candy bar or grabbing a donut. If you want that to happen less often, there's something you can do about it. While preparing foods ahead of time and taking them with you when you're in a hurry is still one of the best strategies, you can make healthy choices just about anywhere if you put your mind to it. The following includes potential grab-and-go options in different situations for meals and snacks.

Breakfast:

- Oatmeal can be found on many fast-food breakfast menus. However, keep in mind that some are loaded with carbs. Check the nutrition information to see if the carbs fit your plan.

- A small fruit and yogurt parfait can fit into most meal plans.

- Try an egg white and cheese breakfast sandwich made with an English muffin, or small breakfast burrito. Steer clear of the biscuit and croissant versions, and skip the bacon and sausage.

Lunch or Dinner:

- Salad bars at the grocery store can make a quick, healthy meal. Just go easy on the mayonnaise-based salads, cheese, and dressing.

- If you opt for fast food, choose the small or junior version of the burger and get a side salad.

- A 6-in. sub turkey sandwich on whole-grain bread and loaded with veggies can fit into most meal plans.

- Many fast-food restaurants offer grilled chicken salad. Choose the light vinaigrette salad dressing and go easy on the cheese and croutons, if included.

- At food courts, 1 slice of a large thin-crust vegetarian pizza fits into most meal plans. Make sure you stick with the thin crust to control your carbs.

Snacks:

- Many grocery stores package a small green salad and a hardboiled egg or some similar combination.

- A 1-oz. string cheese or 2-percent-milk cheddar cheese packet is a good snack fix.

- A granola bar with at least 5 g protein, approximately 17 g of carbohydrate, 2 g or less saturated fat, and approximately 140 calories works for a quick pick-me-up.

- A single-serve tuna (for example, herb and garlic flavor) and cracker snack pack is a good protein snack.

- Try a 6-oz. light or Greek yogurt for a sweeter snack treat.

 DIABETES DECODED

When eating out, remember that the foods are generally much higher in sodium than when you eat at home. Expect the fat and saturated fat to be higher as well.

Additionally, when you have diabetes, it's a smart plan to always carry snacks with you. You never know what can happen when you're traveling or on the go. Always keep a source of carbohydrates to treat hypoglycemia with you in addition to the snacks.

How to Successfully Use Meal Replacements

Beyond the options we've given you previously, you may consider using a meal replacement when on the go. Meal replacements are foods or drinks that can be used to replace all or part of a usual meal. They have proven to be an easy-to-use, effective weight-loss tool for overweight people with diabetes. People with diabetes may benefit from meal replacements that are designed to cause a slower rise in blood glucose and are moderate in carbohydrate content. Meal replacements are also a quick and easy way to get the nutrients you need in place of a complete meal. Because meal replacements are calorie- and portion-controlled, the decision on what and how much you're going to eat is already taken care of; you don't need to make the decision at the time of the meal.

Weight-loss "shakes" and nutrition bars are commonly used as meal replacements, but even the lower-calorie, lower-fat, frozen entrées such as Lean Cuisine, Healthy Choice, or Smart Ones can be used as meal replacements.

When you're on the go and you need something quick, a meal replacement shake or bar may be just the thing. Choose a meal replacement in the following situations:

- Instead of skipping breakfast, grab a shake or bar on your way out the door.

- Use them in place of lunch or dinner, but not both. For instance, you could choose a bar or shake at lunch and a lower-calorie, lower-fat, frozen entrée for dinner.

- Choose a meal replacement instead of choosing a high-fat, salty snack from the vending machine.

- Keep a shake or bar at your desk in case you need to work late or if you miss lunch due to a meeting that goes over time.

The meal replacement product you choose will depend on how you're going to use it. Will it be used for a meal or a snack? If it's a snack, you should choose a product with 150 calories or less. If it will be used for a meal, up to 300 calories is generally fine for most people. Choose meal replacement products that have 2 g or less of saturated fat per serving. The total carbohydrate per serving is also important. Compare the amount to your target carbohydrate amount per meal to make sure it's within your target.

 DIABETES DECODED

> If you just add meal replacement bars or shakes to what you're currently eating, you'll gain weight instead of lose it. The idea is to replace higher-calorie foods with these lower-calorie options.

The Least You Need to Know

- It is possible to successfully lose weight and keep it off long term.
- Don't deprive yourself by going on a diet; give yourself the freedom to choose the foods you want to eat.
- Discovering if you're eating mindlessly and taking steps to become more aware of foods eaten throughout the day may be a useful strategy for weight management.
- Choosing healthful foods when eating on the go can help you control calories and carbohydrates even when you're in a hurry.

CHAPTER 19

Making Your Efforts Pay Off

If you've already started making changes to improve your diabetes management efforts, congratulate yourself. Over time, it's even more rewarding to see results from the work you've been doing. However, what if you're not seeing any benefits even though you're putting in the effort? Without benefits, you won't continue making effort for very long, so it's important to take some time to review your plan and see if something needs to be changed. This chapter takes you through the steps of what you need to do in order to get over any setbacks and gain the benefits you desire.

In This Chapter

- Assessing your meal plan
- Reassessing your weight goal
- The amount of calories burned with exercise
- Recognizing successful weight loss

Meal Planning–Is It Working?

The primary goal of diabetes meal planning is to improve blood glucose control. The meal plan is the foundation for you to achieve your blood glucose targets. Because of this, if your blood glucose has been elevated, the meal plan is the first thing to assess. However, it's important to remember that there are additional factors affecting blood glucose (refer to Chapters 10 and 11 for more information), and sometimes even closely following your meal plan can't change the fact that you need diabetes medication or insulin. So how can you best assess if it's the meal plan that needs to change? Checking your blood glucose both before and after meals helps give you the information you need to identify if the food you eat is contributing to high blood glucose results.

The following is a summary of the blood glucose targets you should be aiming for:

- **Before a meal and fasting:** 80 to 130 mg/dL

- **One to two hours after starting a meal:** Less than 180 mg/dL, with 140 mg/dL or less being considered "normal"

DIABETES DECODED

Even if you already check your blood glucose regularly and know what's happening, you may still need additional testing when assessing your meal plan. If you're not regularly monitoring your blood glucose, you'll need to test it as part of your meal plan assessment process. You really can't tell if your meal plan is working or not working unless you check your blood glucose to find out.

Uncorrected high numbers before a meal set you up for an even higher blood glucose after the meal. While blood glucose monitoring becomes frustrating if it's constantly high, don't throw in the towel and quit testing. Your numbers can improve. On the other hand, if your blood glucose is frequently low and you're not skipping meals or overrestricting your carbohydrates, you may need less diabetes medication. If either one of these issues is happening, contact your medical provider about potential changes to your medication. (More information on blood glucose monitoring is available in Chapter 11.)

Blood Glucose Before Meals

If you take mealtime insulin, you're probably used to checking your blood glucose before meals. However, if you frequently need to take a correction dose of insulin before the meal, something isn't going as planned. When you take diabetes pills or fixed-dose insulin, consistency in carbohydrate intake is key to keeping your blood glucose in target.

While sometimes it's very obvious why the blood glucose is elevated before the meal, sometimes it's not that clear. Therefore, the following table shows you what to consider with your meal planning when your blood glucose is out of range before a meal. Share your blood glucose records with your medical provider, and make sure to include any changes you've made in your meal plan based on your results.

Meal-Planning Considerations Based on Fasting and Before-Meal Blood Glucose Results

Blood Glucose Test	If Your Blood Glucose Is High	If Your Blood Glucose Is Low
Fasting, before breakfast	If blood glucose is greater than 130 but less than 200, eating a small bedtime snack may sometimes lower your fasting blood glucose.	Less than 90 but greater than 70, eating a bedtime snack may help prevent a low blood glucose before breakfast. If your fasting blood glucose is less than 70 more than once, call your medical provider.
Before lunch	You ate too many carbohydrates at breakfast compared to your usual meal plan or the amount of insulin taken.	The amount of carbohydrates you ate at breakfast was too low.
Before dinner	You ate too many carbohydrates at lunch compared to your usual meal plan or the amount of insulin taken.	The amount of carbohydrates you ate at lunch was too low.
Before bed	You ate too many carbohydrates at dinner compared to your usual meal plan or the amount of insulin taken.	The amount of carbohydrates you ate at dinner was too low. If your blood glucose is less than 110, eat a bedtime snack with at least 15 g of carbohydrate. If your blood glucose is less than 80, eat a snack with at least 30 g of carbohydrate.

Notice how the amount of carbohydrates you ate for dinner the night before is not listed as affecting your fasting blood glucose. That's because the effect of the dinner meal is over by the next morning. It's more likely with fasting and before-meal blood glucose you will need an adjustment in your diabetes medication or insulin.

Blood Glucose After Meals

Checking your blood glucose two hours after a meal gives you a much better picture of the effect food has on your blood glucose. Combined with your before-meal results, your after-meal blood glucose results tell you the most about how the food in your particular meal affected your blood glucose. If you've identified your blood glucose is elevated before the meal, even if you eat the right amount of carbohydrates, your blood glucose will likely still be high two hours after the meal. If your blood glucose is on target before the meal and it's elevated after the meal, you probably ate too many carbohydrates at the meal.

Knowing these numbers also helps identify individual responses to certain foods, as well as the overall effects of your meal plan. The following table takes you through the reasons why your blood glucose may be too high or too low after a meal.

Meal-Planning Considerations Based on After-Meal Blood Glucose Results

Blood Glucose Test	If Your Blood Glucose Is High	If Your Blood Glucose Is Low
After breakfast	You ate too many carbohydrates at breakfast compared to your usual meal plan or the amount of insulin taken. If your carbohydrate intake was appropriate, consider changing your food choice—for example, replacing instant oatmeal with cooked rolled oats.	The amount of carbohydrates you ate at breakfast was too low or you skipped the meal. Consider adding carbohydrates or reducing your mealtime insulin dose.
After lunch	You ate too many carbohydrates at lunch compared to your usual meal plan or the amount of insulin taken. Consider taking your lunch to work so you have more control over the carbohydrates included in the meal.	The amount of carbohydrates you ate at lunch was too low or you skipped the meal. Avoid skipping meals by keeping scheduled mealtimes. Eating at least three meals a day, including lunch, helps minimize overeating at dinner.
After dinner	You ate too many carbohydrates at lunch compared to your usual meal plan or the amount of insulin taken. Consider measuring out your food portions to determine if you're eating the right amount of carbohydrates.	The amount of carbohydrates you ate at dinner was too low or you skipped the meal. Eat a snack at bedtime to prevent low blood glucose during the night.

It's important to understand that when you're checking your blood glucose after a meal, the meal most recently eaten has the largest effect on that result.

DIABETES DECODED

If you are referred to a diabetes educator (DE) or registered dietitian/nutritionist (RD/RDN), blood glucose records that include after-meal blood glucose results are almost always requested, though some before-meal blood glucose results may likely be requested as well. DEs and RD/RDNs can then work with you on making changes based on these results. While it's true there are additional factors that can affect your blood glucose, it will be much easier to identify them if you have both before-meal and after-meal blood glucose results.

Reaching Your Weight-Loss Goal

Have you been struggling with weight loss even though you've made changes to your meal plan? It's fairly common for people with both type 1 diabetes and type 2 diabetes to gain weight as their blood glucose improves. For example, you may have experienced weight loss prior to getting diagnosed but, once your hyperglycemia was corrected, found your weight going up. This can be partially due to the fact you are no longer losing extra calories in your urine (in the form of glucose). Certain diabetes medications and insulin can also make it easier to gain weight and more difficult to lose it. So the deck isn't exactly stacked in your favor.

Plus, sometimes the changes in your meal plan are not enough to reach the weight-loss goal you've set for yourself. While most people have room for improvement in the foods they choose, the weight-loss goal itself may be what's to blame. However, if you've been working on changes for a while now, you have a better understanding about the amount of effort it takes to make changes. This makes it a good time to reassess your weight-loss goal and consider if it's realistic or if it needs to be modified. Because realistic goals are more achievable and cause less frustration, setting the right goal may help you get back on track.

Is Your Goal Realistic?

The first step to reassessing your plan is to consider if your weight-loss goal was unrealistic. If so, think about revising it. If you decide to change it, that doesn't mean you're admitting defeat. When you reach your revised goal, you can always revisit your original goal.

For example, say your current goal is to lose 50 pounds by making all of your own meals, to feel better and to improve your diabetes control. There are a few flaws with this plan. First, using an all-or-nothing approach is bound to fail. Second, you may eventually lose 50 pounds, but it's

going to take a while to get there. A goal of losing 50 pounds may be too far off in the future; if you've already lost 5 pounds you are moving toward your goal, but it may still seem unattainable.

Breaking your goal down to a more immediate, stepwise goal and using SMART goal-setting principles to create an action plan may help get you back on track (refer to Chapter 4 for more information about SMART goals). For instance, a smaller weight-loss goal may be appropriate to help build your confidence and maintain your motivation. Here's an example of reframing the goal with that in mind:

> **Original goal:** "Lose 50 pounds by making all my own meals, to feel better and to improve my diabetes control."

> **Revised, more immediate weight-loss goal:** "Lose 10 pounds by limiting the number of times I eat out, to feel better and to improve my diabetes control."

You can then use SMART goals to further refine the goal and determine how you are going to get there, for example: "I will limit the number of times I eat out at restaurants to one time per week or less for the next eight weeks."

DID YOU KNOW?

With weight-loss efforts, 100 percent of people will have a slip or setback. Don't let your setback keep you from continuing your efforts; there are ways around any road-block. Even small changes can lead to success. As Thomas Edison once said, "I have not failed. I've just found 10,000 ways that won't work."

This goal specifies what you're going to do and when. This may or may not be a realistic goal for you personally, depending on how many times you eat out each week. Keep in mind, too, that it may take more than just one action plan to meet your goal, depending on how much the action decreases your calorie intake. By having a goal that's attainable, you're setting yourself up for success not only in the short run but in the long run as well.

Strategies to Stay on Track

Along with having realistic stepwise goals, there are a few other considerations to think about. With any ongoing weight management efforts, there are always ups and downs, with some common issues that come up for almost everyone. Luckily, there are also solutions.

Strategies to get you back on track include the following:

- **Weighing in:** If you're not weighing yourself now, start. For some people, once a week is enough; for others, daily weighing works better.

- **Activity:** Assess your activity level. If you're not where you should be, examine your barriers and think about ways to be more active that minimize the barriers.

- **Support:** Have you tapped into your support system? Do you need additional support? If so, ask for it. Joining a weight-loss group program may also help give you the guidance and support you need. Consider requesting a referral from your medical provider to a local diabetes education program or RD/RDN.

- **Motivation:** Is losing weight important to you? If so, why is it important? List your reasons. How confident are you that you can make the needed changes? Reviewing the importance of losing weight and your confidence level can help you assess if this is really something you want to do and can do.

Number of Calories Burned with Physical Activity

It's much easier to eat calories than to burn them off later. That's why keeping up with your physical activity along with your meal plan remains so important for weight maintenance. However, many people overestimate how many calories they burn with exercise and underestimate the calories they eat. Therefore, it helps to get a better idea of how many calories you're actually burning with various exercises. The following table shows some common 30-minute exercises and how many calories a 155-pound or 185-pound person burns in that time.

Number of Calories Burned in 30 Minutes of Activity

Activity	155-Pound Person	185-Pound Person
Aerobics (water)	149	178
Bicycling (stationery), moderate	260	311
Bowling	112	133
Dancing	205	244
Elliptical trainer	335	400
Gardening	167	200
Golf (carrying clubs)	205	244
Golf (using cart)	130	155
Mowing the lawn (push mower)	205	244
Raking the lawn	149	178

continues

Number of Calories Burned in 30 Minutes of Activity   (continued)

Activity	155-Pound Person	185-Pound Person
Running (5 mph)	298	355
Skiing (cross-country)	298	355
Skiing (downhill)	223	266
Stair-step machine	223	266
Stretching (Hatha yoga)	149	178
Swimming	223	266
Tai Chi	149	178
Tennis	260	311
Walking (3.5 mph)	149	178
Walking (4 mph)	167	200
Walking (4.5 mph)	186	222
Waterskiing	223	266

Adapted from a table originally printed in the July 2004 *issue of the* Harvard Heart Letter.

DIABETES DECODED

If you weigh less than the weight shown on the chart, you will burn fewer calories than listed. On the other hand, if you weigh more than the weight shown on the chart, you will burn more calories for the same activity.

If you're currently maintaining your weight, stepping up the physical activity using these exercises as a guideline may make the difference in your weight-loss efforts. Just remember as you lose weight, your body requires fewer calories, and you'll also burn fewer calories during physical activity than when you started. That's where staying up on and managing your meal plan can help you balance it out.

More than Just the Number on the Scale

When you're monitoring your weight-loss efforts, don't let the scale provide the whole picture. Making positive changes, choosing healthier foods, and improving your fitness all count, too. The scale can seem to be passing judgment at times, telling you whether or not you're worthy. Don't give in to those feelings! What's reflected from the scale is just a number that doesn't mean anything more than that. Plus, everyone hits plateaus during weight loss. If you keep sticking with the plan and keep staying active, the pounds will eventually come off.

At some point, it may not actually be worth losing a few more pounds. For example, say your weight goal was 195 pounds and you've lost 35 pounds but are still 5 pounds short from your goal. If you have it in your head that you have to get below 200 pounds and you can't, you may believe you've failed. However, having to really step up your activity or cut back on your food intake to unrealistic levels to lose the last 5 pounds is probably not worth it. Does it really make a difference? You have already lost weight successfully. Do a few more pounds really mean that much? As far as your health goes, it really doesn't. And who else needs to know about the number on the scale anyway? Celebrate your success!

The Least You Need to Know

- Blood glucose monitoring results can be used to assess how well your meal plan is working.
- Don't assume if your blood glucose stays high that it's somehow your fault. Talk with your medical provider if your numbers are staying high.
- If you're not reaching your weight-loss goal, consider revising it and rethinking your plan.
- The amount of calories you burn with exercise may be less than you think. Increasing your activity is recommended if you aren't meeting your weight-loss goal.
- Recognize when you've been successful with your weight-loss efforts. Don't let the number on the scale be the deciding factor of your success.

Special Considerations: Older Adults and Families

As people are living longer, there is a growing population of people over age 65 in the United States. Because diabetes risk increases with age, over 25 percent of people in this age group have diabetes. There is no one-size-fits-all approach for this age group due to wide range in health status, so individualization is important. In this part, we explain diabetes management considerations unique to older adults related to nutrition, physical activity, and medications. Screening for depression, malnutrition, and dementia is also covered here.

As children in the United States become increasingly overweight and obese, type 2 diabetes in youth (ages 10 to 19) has become a growing concern. When parents have type 2 diabetes, the odds of their children developing diabetes goes up significantly. So in this part, we also discuss nutrition and physical activity recommendations to get the whole family involved in creating a healthy lifestyle to prevent or treat diabetes in children. Creative, nutritious sack lunch ideas are shared, as well as the importance of eating together as a family. We also outline how to create a diabetes plan for your children while at school.

Older Adults and Diabetes

Because older adults have a wide range of physical ability and fitness levels, the term *elderly* won't be used here; instead, we use the term *older adults,* which applies to anyone 65 years and up. While the number of older adults with type 1 diabetes is increasing as people are living longer and healthier with diabetes, the number of people in this age group with type 2 diabetes is significantly higher. So in this chapter, we review unique concerns for older adults related to the care and management of type 2 diabetes. Whether you're reading this chapter for yourself or someone you care about, you'll find some helpful information here.

In This Chapter

- Aging and diabetes
- Diabetes management differences for older adults
- Nutrition issues in older adults
- Maintaining physical activity

Diabetes in Older Adults—What's the Difference?

The oldest in the "baby boomer" population group—those born from 1946 to 1964—are almost 70 years old. Because of the large numbers in this group, they have a significant influence on the country as a whole. Additionally, less people are smoking and health care is more advanced than ever before, so people are living longer. And a Census Bureau report released in 2014 predicted that the number of Americans age 65 and older will almost double by 2050, with adults in this age group accounting for more than one fifth of the total population in the United States at that time. The combination of these factors is having an overall effect on the aging of the country's population. This has been referred to as the "graying of America."

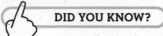

DID YOU KNOW?

According to the CDC, 400,000 people age 65 and older were diagnosed with diabetes in 2012.

Because the risk of type 2 diabetes increases by age 40, older adults may have previously been diagnosed and have been living with diabetes for years, or they may develop diabetes later in life. As a result, the over-65 population has the highest percentage of people with diabetes, at greater than 25 percent.

Are there differences in managing diabetes as an older adult than as a younger adult? The not-so-simple answer is "yes and no." Are you wondering why there isn't a straight answer to that question? Well, the diabetes management strategies actually depend on the individual older adult. Take a minute to think of five people you know that are age 65 and older. Do they work outside the home, participate in regular physical activity, and have the ability to walk up several flights of stairs with ease? Or do they have multiple medical problems, need assistance with routine activities like driving a car or shopping for groceries, and have difficulty standing up after sitting for a while? If you think of the variation in health and fitness levels of these different people, it helps illustrate why diabetes management is not the same across the board for older adults, even if they're the same age. However, it is this variation that makes managing diabetes different for older adults. Out of all the age groups, older adults may be the most diverse in health status, which means individualized treatment plans are critical for the best care.

Factors Affecting Treatment and Targets

Generally, if you are physically and mentally able, as well as willing to self-manage your diabetes, your blood glucose targets will be similar to those for younger adults. However, if there are more risks than benefits to having near-normal blood glucose numbers due to varying health issues, it's reasonable that the targets would be set higher.

Examples of when blood glucose targets might be set higher are the following:

- Poor physical function, such as balance not being good (needing a walker to get around) or low vision (vision changes that are not correctable with glasses or contact lenses)

- *Dementia*

- Multiple medical issues

- Limited life expectancy

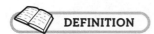 **DEFINITION**

> **Dementia** describes symptoms that affect memory, social skills, thinking, reasoning, judgment, or language. These symptoms in turn affect the ability to perform everyday activities, such as driving a car or balancing a checkbook.

There are several reasons to set your blood glucose targets higher due to these health issues, the main reason being to decrease the chance of hypoglycemia. Hypoglycemia alone can cause life-threatening health risks; in addition, it can lead to falls or other injuries in older adults. Older adults are also more likely to have hypoglycemia unawareness and not experience the early warning signs of a low blood glucose level. With hypoglycemia unawareness, severe hypoglycemia that requires the assistance of others is more likely to occur.

Hypoglycemia in older adults is more likely in the following cases:

- You are taking insulin, glyburide, glipizide, glimeperide, repaglinide, or nateglinide to control blood glucose. Of these medications, insulin and glyburide are the most likely to contribute to hypoglycemia.

- You don't eat meals at scheduled times or you skip meals.

- Your kidneys don't work well—for example, if you've been diagnosed with chronic kidney disease.

- You take five or more medications for various health conditions.

In general, with a higher risk of hypoglycemia, suggested target blood glucose is as follows; check with your doctor about the right targets for you:

- **Fasting or premeal blood glucose:** 90 to 130 mg/dL

- **Bedtime blood glucose:** 100 to 150 mg/dL

- **Target A1C:** Less than 7 percent to between 7 and 7.5 percent, depending on multiple factors (including the amount or type of diabetes medication it takes to keep your blood glucose in the lower targets)

Even if your blood glucose targets are set at a higher level by your doctor than the preceding targets, your blood glucose shouldn't run so high that hyperglycemia causes symptoms or puts you at risk for a medical emergency such as hyperosmolar hyperglycemic syndrome (see Chapter 6 for more on the treatment and prevention of hyperglycemia).

Another important consideration when determining target blood glucose levels is the expected benefit. If complications from diabetes are already in advanced stages or if significant dementia is present, improving blood glucose control to near normal won't have the same benefit as for someone who is newly diagnosed with diabetes, is healthy, and has longer to live. Aside from the risk, it also takes some time to achieve the benefits of good blood glucose control. In this case, lowering high blood pressure may provide more immediate benefits than blood glucose control.

DID YOU KNOW?

Adults 75 years and older have double the number of emergency room visits due to hypoglycemia than those under age 75. If you or a loved one is experiencing hypoglycemia, talk with the appropriate doctor right away; your diabetes medication or insulin might need to be adjusted.

What to Do When You're Feeling Blue

Depression is more common in older adults or in people with diabetes at any age. So the combination of older age and having diabetes makes it much more likely that you'll be dealing with depression at some point. Depression can cause a "snowball effect" with other health problems, potentially leading to poor nutrition status, inactivity, and worsening diabetes control. So it's important to be alert to any signs of depression.

It may not seem obvious that you're depressed, and people you care about may not see what's going on. However, if you feel "low" or "down" and are not enjoying family, friends, or hobbies, you may be depressed. Because it's so common in older adults with diabetes, you should talk with your doctor about being screened for depression. If, along with those issues, you have difficulty sleeping, eating, working, or functioning and it is not getting better, depression is almost certain, don't wait; see your doctor right away. Many treatment options are available, including medication and counseling. Don't think you have to go it all alone; support is available, and treatment options can be effective.

If you're in need of support from family members or other loved ones to deal with diabetes along with feelings of sadness or depression, here are a few things they can do for you:

- Learn more about diabetes and talk about it with you. They can ask about how you are managing diabetes. Listening may be the best support they offer.

- Offer to go on walks; activity helps manage stress, depression, and blood glucose.

- See if you would like reminders for doctor visits, or when to take medication or check blood glucose.

- Ask if they can talk with your health-care team to learn more about how you can help with diabetes management.

- Ask about ways of coping with diabetes and how they can help. Here are some sample questions they can ask you:

> Do you ever feel down or overwhelmed about everything you need to do to manage your diabetes?
>
> Do you have goals to manage your diabetes?
>
> What things get in the way of reaching your goals?
>
> How can I support you in your efforts to manage your diabetes?

Diabetes Medication Complications

The need for individualization of types of medication and appropriate dosing in older adults with diabetes is necessary for the best outcomes. However, there is increased risk of negative side effects from medicine above age 65 due to age-related changes that interfere with the usual way your body clears out the drugs. And when you have multiple medications for various health conditions, the risks—and costs—are even higher. Therefore, it helps to learn more about the medication issues associated with older adults in particular.

Polypharmacy

Polypharmacy sounds like the place you go to pick up your prescriptions rather than a description for multiple medication use, but that's actually what it is. Sometimes several medications are needed just for diabetes management. However, other health conditions like high blood pressure may also require several medications for good control.

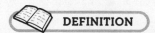 **DEFINITION**

> **Polypharmacy** is a term used to describe multiple different prescription medications for various health conditions being taken at the same time.

Some of the negative consequences of polypharmacy in older adults with diabetes include the following:

- An increased risk of falls and fear of falling

- A significant increase in risk for cognitive impairment

- When seeing multiple doctors for various health conditions, similar medications being prescribed by each doctor, causing duplication

- Drugs interacting with each other, causing different side effects than anticipated

- Increased risk of prescribing and dispensing errors

Plus, if you're taking a number of medications for various medical conditions, it can be difficult to keep track of all the pills. For instance, the pills can add up quickly if you take them for diabetes, high blood pressure, and cholesterol. To help you stay on track, it's a good idea to have a plan in place to take your medications as prescribed.

The following are some suggestions to stay on schedule with your medications; if you don't know when or how often to take a medication, ask your pharmacist or the doctor who prescribed it:

Keep an updated list of all the medications you take. Include prescription, over-the-counter medications, and vitamins or any other supplements you take. It's best to keep this list in your wallet or purse for quick reference. (See Appendix C for a blank medication list you can use to record your medications.)

Take all of your medicines exactly as your doctor tells you. If you're not able to take them for any reason, talk with your doctor to see if something can be changed to make it easier for you.

Keep your medications somewhere in your home that is cool and dry. Bathrooms that get steamy and overly warm are not a good place to store medications.

Fill all of your prescriptions at the same pharmacy, if you can. Make sure they are aware of any allergies you have, and ask them to review your medications and alert you to any issues with your prescriptions.

Use a pill organizer to sort out your medications. Don't mix pills in one container for convenience, especially when you travel. It's easy to get pills mixed up because many look alike. Pill organizers come in various sizes, and some are much easier to open than others. Ask your pharmacist to show you some examples if you're not sure what the best type is for you.

If you have trouble remembering to take your medication, use reminders. You can use "sticky" notes, alarm clocks, or alarms on your cell phone to remind you. You can also center taking your medications around other things you do in your regular routine, such as meals, brushing your teeth, or getting ready for bed.

Ask your doctor about the benefits and risks of taking each prescription. It's important to know why you're taking your medications. If you aren't getting the expected benefit or you aren't comfortable with the risks, let your doctor know.

DIABETES DECODED

If you're a caregiver for an older adult with diabetes, it can be stressful. Therefore, it's important to take care of yourself, too. First, take care of your own health; you need to look out for yourself to be there for the person you care for. Stay physically active, eat well, and follow up with your doctor as needed. If you feel like you're overloaded, when you're asked to commit to additional responsibilities, simply say "No, thank you; I'm overcommitted." And remember, it is okay to ask for and accept help from friends or other family members. Everything does not have to be completed every day. Prioritize and get done what needs to be done; other things can wait. If caregiving gets overwhelming, find someone to talk with or even check out caregiver online resources.

Medication Costs

Even if you are only responsible for a portion of the cost of your medications, it can add up very quickly. And the more medicines you take, the more expensive it gets. If you're having difficulty paying for your prescriptions, ask your pharmacy if you are eligible for any discounts. You can also check with your doctor's office for potential options.

Some available possibilities may help with your prescription drug costs. One potentially significant cost savings is taking generic medication. Ask your doctor if a generic medication can be substituted for a name-brand prescription. Many pharmacies carry generic versions of diabetes medications like metformin, glyburide, and glipizide for $4 for a 30-day supply or $10 for a 90-day supply (total cost). Plus, medications for other health conditions are also available at that same price. Ask your pharmacist if the medications you take are on that low-price generic list. Remember though, even if your pharmacy isn't billing Medicare or other insurance for the medication, you still need a prescription to purchase the pills.

Many of the drug manufacturers also offer prescription assistance through various programs to help with the cost of medications. While some programs are only for people without insurance, some discount card programs are available to people with insurance. For instance, each of the insulin manufacturer companies offer programs to assist with the cost of insulin for people without insurance coverage who meet qualification requirements. Discounts may also be offered for blood glucose test strips and meters. Contact the manufacturer of the medication or product to see if you may qualify. Eligibility criteria are available on each company's website, or you can also contact them by phone.

Differences in Medication Side Effects for Older Adults

There are a few things that doctors consider when prescribing diabetes medication for older adults (see Chapter 10 for more on diabetes medications). The following are some of the special considerations for common diabetes medications.

Metformin: This is the most commonly prescribed diabetes pill, especially when initially starting medication therapy. An important decision-making tool for prescribing metformin is kidney function. A blood test done at a lab can tell if your kidneys are working like they should. The estimated glomerular filtration rate (eGFR) gives the best information on how good of a job your kidneys are doing. The result of the test lets your doctor know whether metformin is safe for you to take. As with any medication, there are benefits and risks. Generally the benefits from metformin outweigh the risks. A plus for older adults is that it doesn't tend to cause hypoglycemia. The downside is that some people end up with gas, bloating, and diarrhea from metformin. So if you already have stomach problems and you're not eating well, it may not be the best option for you. Metformin can also cause some weight loss. While that might be a plus if you're overweight, if you're underweight, additional weight loss wouldn't be a good thing.

Sulfonylureas: These medications have been around for a long time and are available as low-cost generics. The problem with these medications is the higher risk of hypoglycemia. Generally, glipizide and glimepiride can be used safely but might require a lower dose. However, glyburide has a very high risk of hypoglycemia in older adults, so it's not recommended. If you've been prescribed glyburide and are currently taking it, talk with your doctor about trying glipizide or glimepiride instead.

Glinides: Some older adults have a blood glucose pattern where fasting blood glucose numbers are in target range, but after-meal blood glucose levels go way up. The glinide medications repaglinide or nateglinide—which aren't used as frequently as the diabetes pills previously mentioned—may be a good choice when this occurs. These medications are taken just before a meal to bring the blood glucose down after eating, but they don't stay in your system for a long time, making the risk of hypoglycemia lower. Because they are only taken before meals, if a meal is missed or delayed, you won't end up with low blood glucose then either. These medications aren't used as frequently as the diabetes pills previously mentioned.

Eating Right at Any Age

Good nutrition is important for diabetes management and overall health in older adults. Nutrition therapy for diabetes can help prevent hyperglycemia emergencies and minimize the risk of hypoglycemia. Making healthy food choices and getting the nutrients you need also helps you feel better and strengthens your immune system to help you fight off common viruses.

Older adults with diabetes may have additional challenges to healthful eating as compared with younger adults. When nutrient, calorie, and protein needs aren't met, over time, it can lead to *malnutrition,* a common problem for older adults. Poor nutrition status can also contribute to the following in older adults:

- Decline in functional ability

- Muscle and bone loss

- Anemia

- More frequent hospital stays

- Decreased mental alertness

- Delayed wound healing

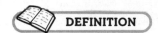 **DEFINITION**

Malnutrition refers to a condition where the body doesn't get enough nutrients for proper function. Malnutrition can be mild or, in extreme cases, life-threatening. Not getting enough nutrients and calories through eating or not being able to properly digest food can lead to malnutrition.

By making an effort to choose the right foods, you can improve your health and have more energy to do things you enjoy.

Addressing Older-Adult Nutrition Concerns

There are challenges to eating healthy at any age. But for older adults, healthy eating becomes more difficult. The following are the different reasons, along with potential solutions:

Appetite generally lessens with age. It may be easier to miss meals due to fewer hunger cues or feeling full quickly after eating a small amount. Some medications can also decrease appetite. Scheduled meal times with reminders can help you get adequate calories, protein, and nutrients.

After years of preparing food for a family, you may be less interested in preparing meals for just one or two people. It's fine to cook larger amounts and freeze portions for later use. That way, you have extra food prepared for when you don't feel like cooking.

You have a limited budget for groceries, making it more difficult to purchase preferred foods. Using store ads to see what's on sale, clipping coupons (only for items you really need), buying store brands instead of name brands, and sticking to your grocery list can increase your cost savings.

It is too physically demanding to shop for groceries and prepare meals, so skipping meals or eating the same convenient foods more often becomes routine. Stocking up on healthy frozen entrées and pantry items for quick meal preparation can help increase the nutritional value of your food choices.

 FOR YOUR SAFETY

> Adaptive cooking utensils such as knives with built-up grips can help people with tremors, neuropathy, arthritis, or poor hand strength stay independent with preparing meals. Special gloves and cutting boards with rubber backing are also available to help prevent injuries from tasks like cutting up vegetables. If you're having difficulty with daily tasks, your doctor can refer you to an occupational therapist who can assess your needs and determine useful kitchen tools to help you stay independent and injury free.

Food safety issues may become more of a problem. Vision and sense of smell are generally not as good in older age, so it becomes more difficult to read expiration dates on labels and easily recognize the smell of spoiled food. Low vision makes meal preparation more challenging as well. To combat this, leftovers should be labeled using a black marker with an expiration date no longer than three days from the first date eaten. When in doubt, throw it out!

Sense of taste decreases in older age, so your food may taste bland and uninteresting. Foods may also taste different than usual. Many medications can cause changes in how foods taste. Adding stronger flavors to food such as salsa, garlic, pepper, and salt-free herb seasoning blends may make foods more enjoyable.

If your teeth are missing or are painful, your food choices may be limited. The texture of the food may not be as appealing if you're restricted to only soft foods and ground meats. Because eating is also a visual experience, creating a colorful plate of food can increase the amount of food you eat.

Sometimes it's difficult to get enough protein. Try to increase protein foods for meals and snacks. If you're not a big meat eater, there are other foods that can be added to your meal plan. For instance, hardboiled eggs can be a good snack, or they can be sliced and added to salads or made into egg salad sandwiches. Also, a 6-ounce serving of Greek yogurt provides the same amount of protein as 2 ounces of meat. If you don't feel like eating a meal, have a liquid nutritional drink or high-protein snack bar. Peanut butter is another great way to add protein while also adding calories at the same time, and including more beans or lentils in your meals (such as salads, soups, and casseroles) helps add protein and fiber at the same time.

You have trouble staying hydrated. Being dehydrated can worsen high blood glucose and cause a hyperglycemic medical emergency. Because thirst isn't a good indicator of actually needing to drink water in older adults, make a plan to drink more fluids throughout the day. Drink a full glass of water when taking medications. Also, keep a glass of water with you when you're at home as a reminder to drink, and include tea, coffee, or water with meals. If getting up in the middle of the night keeps you from drinking water, stop drinking just a few hours before bed, but still drink during the day.

FOR YOUR SAFETY

Are you worried you might not be eating enough? Losing weight without trying may be a sign of poor nutrition status or malnutrition in older adults. If you aren't eating well or are losing weight, ask your doctor for a referral to a registered dietitian/nutritionist (RD or RDN). An RDN experienced in diabetes care can help with ideas to add calories and protein along with meal planning to manage diabetes. And if you'd like to gather some information to take to your doctor, a simple tool is available to assess your nutrition status called the Self-MNA Mini Nutritional Assessment. Designed for people age 65 years and older, you can complete it yourself, or a friend, caregiver, or family member can help you. The form can be downloaded for free from the Nestlé Nutrition Institute at mna-elderly.com/forms/Self_MNA_English_Imperial.pdf.

Getting Enough, But Not Too Much

Because calorie needs decrease with age by 20 to 30 percent while nutrient needs stay the same, it is even more important to choose nutritious foods. In other words, you have to pack the same amount of nutrients into fewer calories than when you were younger. It may be more difficult to get enough of certain vitamins and minerals. Talk with your doctor about the need for a multivitamin supplement. Many people are low in vitamin D, ask your doctor about checking your vitamin D level in your blood.

Overnutrition also contributes to malnourishment in the United States. Eating too much fast food, sweets, chips, snack food, and "junk food" can cause you to gain weight and be malnourished at the same time.

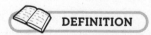

DEFINITION

Overnutrition is caused by eating too many low-nutrient, high-calorie foods and not getting enough activity. Inadequate vitamin, mineral, and fiber intake can occur even with a high volume of calories.

To get the most nutrients in your food choices, keep in mind the following healthy eating principles (see Chapter 12 for the best way to balance your plate):

- Choose a variety of fruit and vegetables in the colors of the rainbow.

- Eat whole grains more often.

- Choose lean protein.

- Include low-fat dairy products.

- Try something new; you never know what you might like, and you can broaden your food options at the same time.

Resources are available to promote healthy eating for older adults. Most communities have home-delivered meal programs, such as Meals on Wheels. Many senior centers also offer on-site meals with balanced food choices; going to the center makes the meal a social time, too.

If you're not eating well and struggling to maintain your weight, it's more important to focus on overall healthy eating rather than being strict with your carbohydrate intake. Make sure to include foods you enjoy eating, as long as you are getting a variety of foods, including protein foods; additional restriction that makes eating less enjoyable isn't necessary.

Overweight Older Adults

Many people with type 2 diabetes are overweight and are insulin resistant. Weight loss is often recommended for people with type 2 diabetes to improve insulin resistance. For older adults, however, there are some concerns about weight loss. A weight loss of 5 to 10 percent of your body weight may be a good idea if you're overweight, but weight loss larger than that is generally not recommended. Some studies have shown that losing weight may actually cause more health problems than being overweight.

The reason for this is that being overweight after the age of 65 may provide extra energy stores during illness and stress. The higher amount of fat stores may also protect from bone loss and developing fractures from osteoporosis. And weight loss that's not intentional is almost always a concern.

That makes activity an important component of any weight-loss plan, especially when you're over age 65. If you don't include activity, you'll generally lose muscle when you lose weight. So it is very important for you to maintain the muscle mass you have by exercising, especially through strength training, along with meal-planning strategies. In fact, this is so important for older adults that no weight-loss plan should be considered without it. (Refer to Chapter 18 for weight management strategies.)

Aging and Activity

The phrase "move it or lose it" definitely applies to physical function. Maintaining the physical function you have is much easier than losing it and trying to gain it back. When combined with healthy eating, physical activity can help you improve your strength, promote a sense of well-being, and improve your diabetes control. Including a variety of physical activity such as leisure activities, aerobic activity, strength training, and balance exercises gives you the most benefit.

Talk with your doctor before you increase your activity to make sure there are no restrictions. If you are having pain or you're not able to move as much as you used to, your doctor can refer you to a physical therapist to assess your range of motion, strength, and endurance. A physical therapist can also recommend assistive devices such as canes, walkers, or shower chairs as needed.

 FOR YOUR SAFETY

If you've been inactive and you're becoming more active, be prepared to treat hypoglycemia by keeping glucose tablets or other forms of carbohydrates with you when exercising away from home. Talk with your doctor about decreasing your medication or insulin if you start experiencing low blood glucose reactions.

Aerobic Exercise Options

Aerobic activity helps keep your heart strong. Aim for 30 minutes at least five days a week. If you can only do 10 minutes at a time, that's okay; do what you can do. Something really is better than nothing!

Examples of aerobic activities include the following:

- **Walking:** For most people, walking is the best activity to start with. You can walk around your neighborhood, at the mall, or on a treadmill. You may want to start walking for about 10 minutes at a time and gradually work up to 30 minutes if you can.

- **Aerobics class:** This type of fun, energizing group exercise is frequently offered as class in the water. Water aerobics are a great way to get the exercise without pressure or strain on your joints. There's also the option of seated chair aerobics, which you can find at some parks and recreation programs or even on DVD. (See Appendix B for exercise resources.)

- **Riding a bike:** You may feel more stable with a three-wheel bike or a stationary bike.

- **Dancing:** However the music inspires you to move is great! You could also consider ballroom dancing classes available through senior centers or your local parks and recreation program.

- **Playing with your grandchildren:** How about a game of hide-and-seek or lawn darts? Your grandchildren will enjoy spending time with you doing any activity where they get to play. Trips to the park are always a hit.

- **Swimming:** If swimming is too much, walking in the shallow end of the pool is also wonderful exercise.

- **Golfing:** If you like to golf, try walking the course for more exercise. If you play 18 holes, you may want to walk the front 9 and use a cart for the back 9.

Strength Training Options

Strength training is even more important as you age. You may think losing muscle as you get older happens to everyone, and that there's nothing you can do about it. Not so; you can maintain and even build muscle at any age! Try to do strengthening exercises at least twice a week.

If you're not sure what counts as strength training, here are some examples:

- Lift "free weights"; soup cans are a good way to get started so you don't choose something that's too heavy. Don't lift more than you're comfortable with.

- Use weight machines at a gym. Get trained on the machines and use the weight that's best for you and your fitness goals.

- Use resistance bands.

- Climb stairs.

- Do exercises that use your own body weight to create resistance. These include activities like push-ups (it's okay to start with wall push-ups) or sit-ups.

- Carry groceries; you can help bag them at the store and lift them in and out of your car.

- Work in your garden hoeing, digging, raking, and so on.

Balance Exercise Options

Including balance exercises in your physical activity plans will help you feel more stable and can help prevent falls. Try to include balance exercises three days a week.

Here are a couple simple balance activities to try:

- Get a good grip on the back of a stable chair. Close your eyes and stand on one foot. Repeat with the other foot.

- After making sure you have a flat, uncluttered floor behind you and you're steady enough on your feet, carefully walk backward and then sideways.

Participating in Tai Chi or yoga classes also help with balance. And to strengthen your legs while improving balance, stand up out of a chair five times in a row each day and build up to 10 repetitions as you can. Once you can do this easily, stand up without "pushing off" with your hands.

The Least You Need to Know

- Diabetes is very common among adults age 65 and older.
- Blood glucose targets and treatment recommendations should not be based on age in the over-65 age group. Physical and mental function, as well as the presence of other health conditions, may be used to help determine blood glucose targets.
- Types of diabetes medications and doses may need to be changed for older adults.
- Healthy eating and physical activity are more important as you age, not less.

Families with Type 2 Diabetes

If you have type 2 diabetes and have children, you may worry that they will also develop type 2 diabetes. While it's true that your kids are at risk, it's also true that there's something you can do about it. If you have children who have already been diagnosed with type 2 diabetes, there are a number of things that you can do to improve their health. This chapter discusses how you can help your children delay or prevent type 2 diabetes and provides tips for keeping your kids healthy and active to manage type 2 diabetes. By learning about the risks and the benefits you can achieve, you're taking the first step on your way to making helpful changes for your whole family.

In This Chapter

- Reducing kids' risk of type 2 diabetes

- Guidance for parents about nutrition and activity

- Diabetes care at school

- Helping teens with type 2

Type 2 Diabetes—It's All in the Family

There are several reasons that type 2 diabetes occurs in families. In previous chapters, it's been mentioned that both genetics and environment play a role in the development of type 2 diabetes. Because you can't change the genes you've inherited and passed on to your children, it may seem like there's not a whole lot you can do. With type 2 diabetes, however, positive changes to your children's environment have a very significant impact on prevention. Even though it's not easy, you as the parent have control over your children's home environment. Making the right changes at home and setting a good foundation can lead to your children maintaining a lifetime of positive health habits.

Kids and Diabetes Risk

Unfortunately, as children and teenagers in the United States are less active and increasingly overweight or obese, type 2 diabetes is becoming more of a problem. This is especially true for kids ages 10 years old and up. According to the National Diabetes Education Program (NDEP), most children and teens diagnosed with type 2 diabetes have a family history of diabetes and are insulin resistant. Just like with adults, type 2 diabetes is more common in some racial and ethnic groups, including African Americans, American Indians, Hispanic/Latino Americans, and Asian and Pacific Islander Americans.

When it comes to genetics, type 2 diabetes is more likely to occur in families than type 1 diabetes. There is a stronger genetic link, so it is more common when parents have type 2 diabetes, their children will also have it. In fact, the ADA states that if you have type 2 diabetes, your children's risk of developing type 2 diabetes is about 1 in 7 if you were diagnosed before age 50 and 1 in 13 if you were diagnosed after age 50. Some scientists think there is an increased risk for children when the parent who has type 2 diabetes is the mother. And when both parents have type 2 diabetes, children's risk is about 1 in 2.

DID YOU KNOW?

Determining your children's risk of type 1 diabetes is a bit more complicated than with type 2 diabetes. According to the ADA, the risk of your children developing type 1 diabetes if you're a man with type 1 diabetes is 1 in 17. If you're a woman with type 1 diabetes and you gave birth to your children before you turned 25, your children's risk is 1 in 25. If you had your children at age 25 or older, your children's risk drops to 1 in 100. However, if you were under age 11 when you developed diabetes, your children's risk of type 1 diabetes doubles. If both parents have type 1 diabetes, the risk varies between 1 in 10 and 1 in 4, depending on other factors.

However, for kids at risk of type 2 diabetes, the strongest factor for actually developing type 2 diabetes is being overweight. Being too heavy increases the amount of fat stores children have. The more fatty tissue there is, the more likely insulin resistance will occur. In addition to weight, being physically inactive is also a significant problem, as regular physical activity helps improve insulin resistance.

Keeping Track of Weight with BMI-for-Age

Because being overweight is such a strong risk factor, helping your child stay at a healthy weight is one of the best things you can do to prevent type 2 diabetes. Therefore, at well-child medical visits, your children's medical provider should monitor their height and weight. It is also recommended that health-care professionals start screening for overweight and obesity in children at 2 years old. One tool used to identify potential weight issues for children is the body mass index (BMI). While BMI is calculated the same for children as it is for adults, it is interpreted differently. BMI is calculated from the height and weight measures and then plotted on the appropriate gender chart.

To calculate children's BMI, use the following:

weight in pounds ÷ height in inches ÷ height in inches again × 703 = BMI

For example, for a child who is 72 pounds and 50 inches tall, you'd get the following BMI:

72 pounds ÷ 50 inches ÷ 50 inches × 703 = 20

Unlike for adults, children and teenagers' BMIs are both age and gender specific and are referred to as BMI-for-age. The reason you shouldn't use the adult BMI table for children is that it doesn't take into account the changes in healthy weight as children grow and gradually lose "baby fat." There are also expected differences in body fat between boys and girls. The BMI-for-age charts are used to assess your children's size and growth pattern, along with how your children's BMI compares among children of the same gender and age. Weight status categories and BMI-for-age percentiles are shown in the following table.

Weight Status Categories for Children BMI-for-Age Percentiles

Weight Status Category	Percentile Range
Underweight	Less than 5th percentile
Healthy weight	5th to less than 85th percentile
Overweight	85th percentile to less than 95th percentile
Obese	Equal or greater than the 95th percentile

If your children haven't had a well-child visit lately and you'd like to calculate BMI, use the following to get an accurate height and weight in order to calculate your children's BMI.

Accurately Measuring a Child's Height:

1. Ensure your child is not wearing shoes or any bulky clothing. Also, make sure your child's hair is flat, free of hair ornaments, and not placed in a hairstyle that might affect the measurement.

2. Have your child stand on the floor where there isn't any carpet and against a flat surface, such as a wall without molding. Have your child stand with his feet flat and together, his heels against the wall. Ensure his legs are straight, his arms are at his sides, and his shoulders are level. If possible, his head, shoulders, and buttocks should be touching the wall.

3. Ask your child to look straight out and ahead, not up or down.

4. Take the measurement using something flat and even for a headpiece (for example, a ruler) to form a right angle with the wall. Lower the piece until it firmly touches the crown (top) of your child's head. Make sure your eyes are at the same level as the piece you are using to measure.

5. Lightly mark where the bottom of the headpiece meets the wall.

6. Use a metal measuring tape to measure from the floor up to the mark on the wall to determine the height measurement.

7. Record the height to the nearest one-eighth inch.

Accurately Measuring a Child's Weight:

1. Use a digital bathroom scale for accuracy. Place the scale on a flat floor, such as tile or wood, not carpet.

2. Make sure your child is wearing lightweight clothing and no shoes.

3. Have your child stand with both feet in the center of the scale.

4. Record the weight to the nearest decimal—for example, 45.1 pounds.

To find out your child's BMI-for-age percentile, charts can be found online at the following (make sure you use the correct gender chart):

- **BMI percentile chart for girls ages 2 to 20:** cdc.gov/growthcharts/data/set2clinical/cj41l074.pdf

- **BMI percentile chart for boys ages 2 to 20:** cdc.gov/growthcharts/data/set2clinical/cj41l073.pdf

DIABETES DECODED

These BMI-for-age charts are used for screening, not diagnosis. If the BMI-for-age indicates overweight status, your children's medical provider may perform additional assessments.

Testing for Type 2

Screening for type 2 diabetes should begin at 10 years old or at the onset of puberty, whichever is sooner. However, if your children have symptoms of diabetes, have them tested for diabetes right away. Symptoms of diabetes in children are similar to adults: feeling tired, increased thirst, having to urinate more often, unexplained weight loss, blurry vision, slow healing of cuts or wounds, and urinary tract infections (burning when urinating). If your child doesn't have symptoms and you're not sure if you should request a test for type 2 diabetes, the primary testing criteria is that your children are overweight, meaning they have a BMI greater than the 85th percentile for their age and gender or weight for a height greater than the 85th percentile for their age and gender. They must also have any two of the following risk factors:

- A family history of type 2 diabetes in either a first-degree relative (a parent, brother, or sister), or a second-degree relative (a grandparent, aunt, or uncle)

- Race/ethnicity (being American Indian, African American, Hispanic/Latino, Asian American, or Pacific Islander)

- Signs of insulin resistance or conditions associated with insulin resistance (for example, *acanthosis nigricans,* high blood pressure, high cholesterol or triglycerides, *polycystic ovary syndrome [PCOS],* or low birth weight)

- If the mother had type 2 diabetes or gestational diabetes during the pregnancy with this child

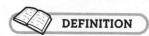

DEFINITION

Acanthosis nigricans is a skin condition that usually occurs in skin folds around the neck, armpits, or groin. Skin becomes thickened, and a dark, velvety discoloration occurs. Children who develop this skin condition are at higher risk of having insulin resistance, and therefore developing type 2 diabetes.

Polycystic ovary syndrome (PCOS) occurs in women and teenage girls when reproductive hormones are out of balance. PCOS causes cysts to form on the ovaries and makes menstrual periods become infrequent or stop altogether. Acne and excess facial hair growth can also occur. PCOS is linked with insulin resistance and type 2 diabetes.

Your child's medical provider may order a fasting blood glucose test, an A1C test, or both to screen for type 2 diabetes. There also may be a reason to check for diabetes even if your child doesn't meet all the criteria, such as having a related health condition. If you have concerns, talk with your child's medical provider.

Parents: How to Help Your Kids

Children learn habits, both good and bad, from their parents. Even though it doesn't always seem like it, what you do and say in front of your kids really does make a difference. They often observe more than you think they do. You may be reminded of that occasionally when you hear your children repeat something you've recently said, often in the most embarrassing way and at the most embarrassing time! The good news is that if you're committed to making changes, your kids will be, too. However, it's important to be consistent and stick with it, even if you don't see immediate results.

Parents Are Role Models

As a parent, your children look to you for guidance and as an example of how to behave and act around others. This is true for eating and physical activity behaviors as well. For instance, if you avoid eating anything green and sit on the couch with remote in hand every evening, your children observe this behavior. It would then be very difficult to get your children to eat green vegetables if you never eat them. And because surfing the channels isn't really a sport, your inactivity can lead to your children's inactivity. So it's important to recognize that you are a role model and that "do as I say but not as I do" is not an effective strategy in creating positive health changes for your family. Whatever healthy eating and activity changes you feel your child should make, you'll need to commit to making those changes, too.

Ellyn Satter is an RDN and family therapist who is well-known for her guidance for parents on child and family eating behaviors (see Appendix B for more information). A key principle from her guidelines is the division of responsibility for feeding between parents and children. For children who are toddlers on up to teens, she shares the following:

- Parents are responsible for what, when, and where the children eat.

- Children are responsible for how much and whether to eat.

So what does this mean for you as a parent in everyday situations? Here's our loose interpretation of Satter's words.

What: The "what" means the parents prepare and offer healthy food choices, but the children have the final say in whether they eat those foods. Parents have to be consistent in offering foods even if the children aren't currently choosing them. It may take multiple offers of spinach, for instance, before your children actually choose to eat spinach. But if you consistently choose to eat and enjoy spinach, eventually your child will, too. Strategies that force kids to eat, such as making your children sit at the table until they eat all of their vegetables, do not work. The children can always outlast the parents. And then what is the lesson learned? Probably not the enjoyment of those vegetables!

The opposite is true for so-called "bad" foods. If these foods are overly restricted or never allowed, it can backfire on you even though you have great intentions. Your kids will tend to want any restricted foods more—for instance, sweets and desserts. To counter this, offering everyone in the family a small portion of dessert with some meals can take away the feeling that sweets are totally off-limits. If you allow your child to eat sweets occasionally, sweets won't seem like such a big deal when they are available away from home.

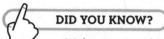

DID YOU KNOW?

Without too much interference and the right opportunities, children will eat the amount they need. It's the children's job to learn to eat foods eaten by the rest of the family and behave appropriately during meals.

When: The "when" means having scheduled mealtimes and snacktimes. For example, having a snack right after school is an ideal time; however, having a snack 20 minutes before dinner is served is not. It's important that your children know and understand when snack and mealtimes are. Having a family meal time observed where everyone sits down to eat together is important. This is a time to share what's happened during the day and gives you the opportunity to really listen to your children. Having meals together also helps children by learning how they should act during meals and what behavior is acceptable at the table. By watching you, they can learn the way they should act. If your children or teens choose not to eat what's offered at snacktime and/or mealtime, that's fine. However, it's important to not offer other foods in place of what they chose not to eat. Only water should be offered between meals and scheduled snacks.

If your children take insulin, mealtime insulin can be given immediately after the meal based on the amount of carbohydrates actually eaten. If your children don't eat, you don't give them the mealtime insulin. This will help prevent hypoglycemia. A carbohydrate source (such as 4 ounces of juice) should still be available to your child if hypoglycemia occurs. Regular blood glucose monitoring can also help prevent low blood glucose.

Where: The "where" means the place the snacks and meals are eaten. Snacking or eating meals in front of the television, while playing games on the computer, or in the children's bedrooms can lead to overeating or eating inappropriate food choices. A recommended place for snacks and meals would be in the kitchen or dining room. You can make it a household rule that snacks are not allowed in a bedroom or other rooms of the house; this helps avoid distractions while eating and helps children focus on the enjoyment of the food. Meals should be eaten while sitting at the table with the television and mobile devices (cell phones, tablets, and so on) turned off. This is a good idea for after-school snacks as well.

Controlling Your Environment

To summarize wellness goals for kids, the Consortium to Lower Obesity in Chicago Children came up with a way to easily remember what to do. It's called *5-4-3-2-1 Go!*, which represents the following:

- 5 servings of fruits and vegetables a day
- 4 servings of water a day
- 3 servings of low-fat dairy a day
- 2 or less hours of screen time a day (includes computer, television, and video games)
- 1 or more hours of physical activity a day

Something that's been added by others after the original 5-4-3-2-1 Go! development is "+10," representing the number of hours of sleep. School-age children need about 10 hours of sleep each night, while teens usually need between 8 and 9 hours a night.

These guidelines can help you make decisions about your home environment along with your usual routine. Here are some tips to meet these guidelines:

- Have set times for the whole family for eating meals and snacks, and when to go to bed.
- Have plenty of nonstarchy veggies such as carrots, celery, salad greens, cherry tomatoes, cucumbers, and bell peppers available and ready to eat. Veggies can be added to any snack or meal if your kids (or you) are still hungry after eating.
- Keep fruit on hand for your kids to grab in place of sweets or chips. This ensures they are getting fiber, vitamins, and other nutrients instead of "empty calories."
- Offer low-fat or nonfat milk or water with meals.
- Choose to leave the empty-calorie snack foods out of your pantry. If you choose to include them, do so less often and in smaller portions.
- Leave televisions out of your children's or teens' room. This is also a good idea for tablets, laptops, or handheld games.
- Set limits on screen time, but not reading, drawing, or using the computer for homework.

- Choose not to offer sweets as a reward. Words of praise go a long way with kids and teens. For younger children, earning stickers for good behavior is a fun way to make them feel recognized.

- Create opportunities for your children to be active, but don't force them to be active. That can backfire, just like making them eat vegetables!

Kids and teens actually thrive on structure, but if you haven't had set routines in your home up until now, change doesn't happen overnight. If you stick with it, you'll find it's well worth it in the long run.

 DID YOU KNOW?

The ADA has information and resources for parents and kids with diabetes available at diabetes.org/families.

How Words Make a Difference

Being a parent is hard work. Learning to say and do things differently than what you heard from your parents growing up is tough. Phrases like "you'd better clean your plate," "if you don't eat your dinner, you won't get dessert," and even "just take one more bite, then you can leave the table" don't seem that negative, but they can be. The other thing about these phrases is that they don't actually yield the results you want.

What should you say instead? Here are some examples of common statements and what you can replace them with:

"Just try one bite for me." *Instead, try: "These berries are sweet and juicy."* This describes the food and what they can expect if they eat it instead of having them earn your approval by eating a certain food.

"Your brother cleaned his whole plate, why can't you?" *Instead, try: "Do you feel full?"* You may be unintentionally teaching your children to ignore feelings of fullness by telling them to eat everything on their plate. Encouraging them to explain how they feel physically, such as "my tummy's full right now" may help them be more in tune to their hunger and fullness.

"That didn't taste so bad, did it?" *Instead, try: "Did you like that?"* When your children try new food, the former statement tells them they made a bad decision about not wanting the food. If they try and don't like the food, it is difficult to come up with an appropriate comment. A simple observation that could be used, whether they like it or not, is "People like different foods, don't they?"

Get Active, Play Active!

Physical activity is important for not only children, but adults as well. Add in some family fun to get both you and your kids moving more. Many people say they don't have time for physical activity, but somehow they have time for their favorite television shows and computer games. If that sounds familiar, you may be amazed at just how much time you have when you turn off the television! Plan for family activity time throughout the week, and mark your chosen times on the calendar to track your progress.

To combat those times when your children need to occupy themselves with something besides the television after school, sit down with your children and help them come up with a list of after-school activities. Examples are walking the dog or playing with the dog in the backyard, riding their bikes, helping make dinner, playing active video games (such as active sports games or ones with dancing), or letting them create their own dance moves to their favorite music. Once they make the list, keep it in plain sight so they can refer to it when they get home. Make your children responsible for their own boredom. That way, they will come up with something to do, and you don't have to give in to turning on the television. You can also have your kids help out with vacuuming, gardening, mowing the lawn, and raking leaves after school or on the weekends.

Outdoor family activities such as going to the park, playing catch in the yard, playing lawn games, and walking the dog often go by the wayside during bad weather months. It is good to have a contingency plan to continue with activity during the winter. Try out an exercise video that the whole family might enjoy, look for an indoor swimming pool in your area, play "dance off" with your kids to see who can come up with the funniest or best dance moves, join a gym, or walk at the mall together. You can even look into fitness classes, which are typically indoors and a great way for kids to move more. Ask your children what they might be interested in, such as swimming, gymnastics, tennis, dance, or martial arts.

 DIABETES DECODED

While you're waiting for your children to get out of a class, you can get your own workout by taking a walk outside or going up and down nearby stairs. The same is true if your child is active in school sports. If you normally just drop them off and pick them up, stay and take a walk around the field during practice.

Dealing with Type 2 Outside the Home

Kids with type 2 diabetes are not just mini-adults with diabetes. There are unique challenges, like helping them eat enough to meet nutrient needs for growth and development without eating too much. By setting the right examples at home, kids make better decisions when they're away from home. But while you have control over the home environment, it's a different story when they are away from home. Because school makes up the largest amount of time your children are away from home, it's good to be involved in what goes on there. By talking to the right people at your children's school, you can be assured a successful plan is in place. Plus, you can create healthy snacks and school lunches to help your children get the nutrients they need without all the extra calories.

Creating a Plan

When it comes to helping your children at school, the ADA has a number of resources for diabetes care at school available at diabetes.org/living-with-diabetes/parents-and-kids/diabetes-care-at-school/. These "Safe at School" resources include information on how to develop written plans with the school to address specific needs for your children in certain situations, including individualized health plans and 504 plans. The 504 plan is an agreement that ensures your children with diabetes have the same access to education as other students. It helps to avoid misunderstandings between the students, parents, and school staff.

When developing the written plan with the school, it helps to outline the roles and responsibilities that everyone has in helping your children with diabetes at school. Examples of situations that might need to be addressed in your child's plan include the following:

- Making sure that school staff, who have direct contact with your child, are trained to recognize high and low blood glucose signs and symptoms and understand the actions they need to take. This includes teachers, coaches, and bus drivers, if applicable.

- Ensuring that appropriate staff members are trained to check blood glucose and administer insulin or glucagon, if needed.

- Letting your children test their blood glucose and respond with the appropriate action—for example, treating a low blood glucose with glucose tablets.

- Allowing additional excused absences for medical appointments, if necessary.

 FOR YOUR SAFETY

If your children with type 2 diabetes are taking diabetes medication or insulin, it is important to understand the signs, symptoms, and treatment of hypoglycemia. Symptoms of hypoglycemia may be a bit different in children than in adults. Symptoms for children include blurry vision or trouble focusing, headache, being cranky or moody, a lack of coordination, crying for no reason, shaking, sweating, confusion, and bad dreams or restless sleep. Make sure that people who spend time around your children are familiar with these symptoms, including your children's friends and key adults at school.

When parents and school staff work together toward keeping your children with diabetes healthy while optimizing learning and education, it's a win-win situation. Remember, being an advocate for your children shouldn't be focused on winning or losing. Disagreements between you and school personnel may happen. If so, a good first step is to educate them about your children's situation and if that doesn't work, plan to thoughtfully negotiate when something needs to be changed.

Healthy Sack Lunch and Snack Ideas

Out of ideas for your kids' sack lunch? It's easy to get stuck in a rut when dealing with what children will eat. The same old sandwich and piece of fruit get a bit boring. Keep it interesting with a bit of variety. Here are a few lunch suggestions:

Bake part of your dinner meal in muffin cups for perfect-size lunch portions. For example, a brown rice, broccoli, and chicken casserole made with low-fat cream of mushroom soup, topped with 2-percent-milk cheddar cheese is great for lunch. You can heat the leftovers to 165°F and put them in an insulated food jar in the morning for your children to take for lunch. Add a serving of unsweetened applesauce and light yogurt for a complete meal.

Make sandwiches with mini whole-wheat bagels and slices of 2-percent-milk cheese. Ask your children to choose veggies in the color of a rainbow (at least three) and add slices of the veggie to the sandwich (for example, purple cabbage, spinach, and yellow pepper). You can also include some apple slices with flavored reduced-fat cream cheese spread along with some carrots and celery sticks as sides.

Fix chili with beans. You can include separate small snack bags or reusable containers with toppings such as shredded low-fat cheese; crumbled multigrain crackers or tortilla chips; and finely chopped veggies like broccoli, red peppers, and green onion. Add a mandarin orange and a few vanilla wafer cookies to make a balanced lunch.

Use a fun-shaped cookie cutter to create a special sandwich. Choose a whole-grain bread, such as 100 percent whole wheat, and a filling like a chopped hardboiled egg with light mayonnaise. You can add some sugar snap peas and cherry tomatoes with a low-fat dip and a sugar-free pudding cup.

Use up leftovers by making quesadillas. If you have rotisserie chicken for dinner, add chicken with low-fat cheese, veggies of your children's choice, and a bit of salsa to a tortilla. Include sliced pears and cottage cheese as sides.

Make a homemade version of Lunchables with low-fat cheese slices, whole-grain crackers, and lower-sodium lunch meat. You can include sliced cucumbers and shredded carrots for toppings. Add a whole-grain granola or snack bar with approximately 15 g of carbohydrate and a small banana to complete the meal.

Whatever you're thinking for your children's lunch, involve your children in choosing foods to include in lunches. Younger children can participate in making their lunches, while older ones can make their own with the ingredients you select together. Beverages should be nonfat or low-fat milk and water only. While up to 6 ounces of 100 percent fruit juice can be included daily, sugary beverages (such as regular soda) should be nixed; they are a leading cause of obesity in children and can lead to high blood glucose. The ADA recommends avoiding sugary beverages completely.

 FOR YOUR SAFETY

> To keep your children's sack lunch safe to eat, remember to keep hot foods hot and cold foods cold. Using an insulated lunch bag with a freezer ice pack can keep foods cold until your child is ready to eat. Cold foods should be kept under 40°F for safety. If you'd like to include hot foods like soup or chili, invest in a good-quality thermos or insulated food jar for more solid foods. There are a number of newer products available that will keep food hot until lunchtime. If you're using the previous night's leftovers, heat the food to 165 F before placing in the container. Hot foods should stay at or above 140 F to keep bacteria at bay. Also, remember to wash any reusable containers with soap and water and to let them air-dry after each use.

When it comes to snacks, they play an important role in meeting nutrition needs. Therefore, don't leave them out, even if your children are overweight. Eating an after-school snack may help prevent overeating at dinner. It may also help prevent a low blood glucose level if your children take diabetes medication. You can have nutritious snacks available that you select and want to offer and then allow your children to choose between them. For instance, instead of saying "Would you like an orange for your snack?" ask, "Would you rather have an orange or a (light) yogurt for your snack?"

Here are some snack ideas for school-age children with type 2 diabetes that contain approximately 15 g of carbohydrate or 1 carbohydrate choice:

- 3 graham cracker squares and 1 TB. peanut butter
- 4 oz. sugar-free pudding cup
- 4 oz. 100 percent fruit juice mixed with 4 oz. sparkling water and 1 oz. string cheese
- Turkey roll-up: 1 to 2 slices of turkey on a small 6-in. tortilla with lettuce and a dab of mustard and/or light mayonnaise
- $^{1}/_{2}$ whole-grain English muffin topped with spaghetti sauce and low-fat cheese, topped with a sliced tomato and chopped bell peppers
- 8-oz. glass nonfat milk or soy milk with cucumber slices and cherry tomatoes

- Single serving fruit cup with $^1/_4$ cup low-fat cottage cheese

- 3 cups air-popped or light microwave popcorn

- 6 oz. light yogurt

- Hardboiled egg with 8 whole-grain crackers (check the label for carbohydrate content)

- 1 cup vegetable soup

- Small apple with 1 TB. almond butter

- Carrot and celery sticks (or any nonstarchy veggies) with 2 TB. hummus and 8 whole-grain crackers (check the label for carbohydrate content)

 DIABETES DECODED

Children's nutrient and calorie needs vary significantly depending on age, gender, activity level, and weight goals. Check with your medical provider or RDN about the appropriate portions to meet your children's nutrition needs.

Teens and Diabetes

Teenagers face some unique situations when it comes to diabetes. If you have a teenager with diabetes, think of all the additional challenges that present themselves on a daily basis. While teens have a lot going on already, diabetes may seem like too much to handle. Physical changes happen quickly at this age and can make diabetes management even more complex. Going through puberty and having hormone fluctuations isn't easy when you don't have diabetes, let alone when you do. Hormones may cause feelings of stress or irritability. Add blood glucose variations—highs and lows—to that and you may find those mood swings getting out of control. It's a good idea to have your teens check their blood glucose to see what's happening when they feel especially stressed or upset. Sometimes the blood glucose may be driving the emotions. If it's high or low when they check, it can help them remember to consider blood glucose as a contributing factor for their feelings.

Teens with diabetes are also exposed to all the same pressure as other teens, but the consequences can be more detrimental for them. Make sure to talk with your teenager about smoking, alcohol use, and drugs. They will listen to you and be much more likely to come to you with concerns if you are open and actively listen to them.

DIABETES DECODED

Girls with diabetes may also find that blood glucose levels fluctuate with their menstrual cycle. Blood glucose may go up or down just prior to, or during, their period. This is caused by hormone changes.

The Least You Need to Know

- Being overweight is the biggest risk factor for developing type 2 diabetes in kids who are at risk.
- Helping your children establish healthy eating and physical activity habits is a good strategy for both prevention and management of type 2 diabetes.
- Parents are role models. You need to commit to making the positive lifestyle changes you'd like your children to make.
- When creating a plan, it helps to outline the roles and responsibilities that everyone has in helping your children with diabetes at school.
- With teens, consider blood glucose as a contributing factor for their feelings.

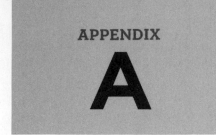
Glossary

A1C   Also called *glycosylated hemoglobin, hemoglobin A1C,* and *HbA1c,* a blood test used to measure diabetes control. It provides an estimate of average blood glucose over two to three months.

AADE7   A framework developed by the American Association of Diabetes Educators of seven self-care skills to effectively manage diabetes. It includes healthy eating, being active, monitoring, taking medication, problem solving, reducing risks, and healthy coping.

acanthosis nigricans   A skin condition that usually occurs in skin folds around the neck, armpits, or groin. Skin becomes thickened, and a dark, velvety discoloration occurs. Children who develop this skin condition are at higher risk of having insulin resistance and therefore developing type 2 diabetes.

acceptable daily intake (ADI)   A safety standard set by the FDA for no-calorie sweeteners. The ADI has a 100-fold safety factor; it is 100 times less than the amount of an ingredient that can be safely consumed on a daily basis over a lifetime without risk or "no adverse effect."

acute   A condition with abrupt onset and rapid progression.

aerobic exercise   Sustained exercise with adequate fuel and oxygen.

alpha cells   Cells in the pancreas that make glucagon.

amino acids   The building blocks of protein.

amylin   A hormone produced in the beta cells of the pancreas that works with insulin to lower blood glucose after meals.

antioxidant   A substance that protects the body's cells from damage caused by oxygenation. Vitamin C and vitamin E are examples of antioxidants.

autoantibodies   Proteins produced by the immune system that react to their own cells and tissues in autoimmune disease.

autoimmune disease   A disease that causes the body's immune system to assault its own tissues. The immune system is designed to seek out and destroy invaders of the body to provide protection from bacteria, viruses, and cancer. Damage is caused when the immune system becomes misdirected and attacks the body tissues it is designed to protect. *See also* type 1 diabetes.

beta cells   Cells in the pancreas that make insulin.

body mass index (BMI)   An estimated measure of body fat based on height and weight that's used to classify people as underweight, normal, overweight, or obese. It is used as a predictor for health risks.

carbohydrates   Also known as carbs, one of the main components in food. Carbohydrates are broken down into glucose, which the body uses for energy.

central nervous system   The part of the nervous system that is comprised of the spinal cord and brain. It's the part of the nervous system that coordinates the activity of the entire nervous system, which includes the peripheral nervous system and central nervous system. The central nervous system needs glucose, generated from carbohydrates, to use for fuel.

cholesterol   A waxy substance made in the body by the liver, which circulates it through the blood. Dietary cholesterol is found in animal foods, such as meat, poultry, and full-fat dairy products. Your liver produces more cholesterol when you eat a diet high in saturated and trans fats.

chronic   A disease or condition that is persistent and long lasting. A chronic disease is generally not preventable by a vaccine or curable with medical treatment, so the goal of treatment is to manage it. Some chronic diseases like diabetes can be well managed and controlled.

cystic fibrosis–related diabetes   A type of diabetes caused by cystic fibrosis. Insulin is required for treatment due to scarring in the pancreas.

dementia   Describes symptoms that affect memory, social skills, thinking, reasoning, judgment, or language. These symptoms in turn affect the ability to perform everyday activities, such as driving a car or balancing a checkbook.

diabetes educator   A trained health-care professional who helps people with diabetes learn self-care skills, achieve behavior change goals, and improve their health status.

diabetic ketoacidosis (DKA)   A life-threatening condition that affects people with type 1 diabetes. It happens when there is not enough insulin for the body to use the glucose in the blood as fuel; instead, fat becomes the fuel source. As fat is broken down, ketones are produced as a waste product. High levels of ketones in the blood become toxic. DKA is caused by missed or inadequate insulin doses.

diabetic nephropathy   Kidney damage caused by diabetes. It is a long-term complication of diabetes that can lead to kidney failure.

diabetic retinopathy   A complication of diabetes that affects the eyes. It causes progressive damage to the retina and can lead to blindness.

diastolic blood pressure   The lower number on the blood pressure reading, which represents the pressure when the heart is at rest.

dietary fiber   An indigestible carbohydrate found in plant foods. There are two main types: water soluble and insoluble.

dietary supplement   A product people take in pill, liquid, or powder form to increase the nutritional value of their usual diet. Dietary ingredients used in supplements are vitamins, minerals, and herbs, among others.

DPP-4 (dipeptidyl peptidase-4)   An enzyme that breaks down the GLP-1 hormone. DPP-4 inhibitors are medications used to manage type 2 diabetes.

drug class   A group of medications with comparable chemical structure that work in a similar way. Typically, they are used to treat the same health issue.

endocrine system   A collection of glands that regulates metabolism, reproduction, growth, mood, sleep, and other bodily functions.

endocrinologist   A physician who specializes in the treatment of the endocrine system. Some endocrinologists are diabetes specialists.

fasting blood glucose   The amount of glucose in the blood after not eating for at least eight hours (usually overnight).

Food and Drug Administration (FDA)   The federal agency that regulates food ingredients, food labels, dietary supplements, and medications.

gene mutation   A permanent alteration in the DNA sequence of a gene. Gene mutations can be inherited from one or both parents, or they can be acquired. Acquired mutations happen in the DNA of cells during a person's lifetime and are not passed on to the next generation. Changes can be triggered by environmental factors such as ultraviolet radiation from the sun or DNA errors as it copies itself as cells divide. Type 1 and type 2 diabetes result from genetic mutations and environmental triggers.

generics   Drugs that are equivalent in dosage and content to brand-name drugs but not marketed under the brand name in order to be lower in cost. Instead, they are referred to by the chemical name. Generics must meet FDA standards demonstrating they are equivalent to the original brand-name medication before they are allowed on the market.

gestational diabetes   Diabetes that is first diagnosed during pregnancy. The blood glucose usually returns to normal after the pregnancy.

GLP-1 (glucagonlike peptide-1)   One of the incretin hormones that increases insulin, decreases glucagon, and delays stomach emptying following a meal.

glucagon   A hormone made by the alpha cells of the pancreas that regulates glucose production in the liver. To keep blood glucose from going too low, glucagon is released at times when you're not eating, such as overnight.

glucose toxicity   A "vicious cycle" in which hyperglycemia itself contributes to even higher blood glucose levels. The hyperglycemia causes injury to the beta cells of the pancreas, causing less insulin production and then more insulin resistance. It is reversible by getting the blood glucose levels under control.

glycogen   The main source of stored carbohydrates in the body. When glucose is not needed for energy, it is converted to glycogen and stored mainly in the liver and muscles.

heart disease   A condition related to the narrowing and blockage of blood vessels that can result in chest pain, heart attack, or stroke.

hemoglobin   A protein found in red blood cells that carries oxygen in the blood.

hormones   Compounds produced by glands in the endocrine system that send a chemical message, which affects the functions of the receptive organs or tissues.

hyperglycemia   A high level of glucose in the blood.

hyperosmolor hyperglycemic state   A serious condition that develops when severe dehydration contributes to extreme hyperglycemia without the presence of ketones. This potentially life-threatening emergency is most common in older adults with type 2 diabetes.

hypertension   High blood pressure.

hypoglycemia   A low blood glucose level.

hypoglycemia unawareness   When a person with diabetes doesn't feel the early warning signs of low blood glucose, such as being dizzy, shaky, hungry, or irritable. People with hypoglycemia unawareness are more likely to experience severe consequences like stupor, seizures, or loss of consciousness without warning. This condition is more common in people with a history of chronic hypoglycemia, such as those with longstanding type 1 diabetes or those with type 2 diabetes who are taking certain diabetes medications (including insulin) that can contribute to low blood sugar.

incretin   A hormone that increases the insulin response after a meal. The two main incretins are glucagon-like peptide-1 (GLP-1) and glucose-dependent insulinotropic polypeptide (GIP).

insulin   A hormone produced by the pancreas that helps the body control blood glucose and store fat.

insulin resistance   When cells are not able to respond normally to insulin, making it more difficult for glucose in the blood to enter the cells.

ketones   Substances produced during the breakdown of fat for energy.

lactic acidosis   A serious condition caused by lactic acid building up to high levels in the blood.

lacto-ovo vegetarian   A vegetarian who eats eggs and dairy.

lacto-vegetarian   A vegetarian who eats dairy products.

latent autoimmune diabetes in adults (LADA)   A type of diabetes diagnosed in adults that is similar to type 1 diabetes but is often misdiagnosed and treated as type 2 diabetes.

lipid panel   A blood test that measures triglycerides, total cholesterol, LDL cholesterol, and HDL cholesterol. High levels of lipids in the blood increase risk of heart disease.

long-term diabetes complications   Conditions that occur gradually when blood glucose has not been well managed over a period of years. The extra glucose traveling in the blood causes damage to both small and large blood vessels, as well as the nerves. Examples of long-term complications include blindness (damage to the retina in the eye), kidney failure, heart disease, and neuropathy (nerve damage causing numbness, tingling, and pain in the feet).

low-calorie sweetener   Also known as *sugar alcohol* or *sugar replacer,* a reduced-calorie carbohydrate used in sugar-free food products.

macrovascular complications   Diabetes complications involving the large blood vessels in the body. Heart disease, stroke, and peripheral artery disease are macrovascular complications.

malnutrition   A condition where the body doesn't get enough nutrients for proper function. Malnutrition can be mild or, in extreme cases, life-threatening. Not getting enough nutrients and calories through eating or not being able to properly digest food can lead to malnutrition.

maturity-onset diabetes of the young (MODY)   A less common form of diabetes that is more like type 2 diabetes but may be confused with type 1 diabetes initially because it's usually diagnosed in children, teens, and young adults.

Mediterranean diet   A traditional eating pattern that reflects the style of eating in countries along the shores of the Mediterranean Sea. The typical eating pattern includes fruit, whole grains, fish, and a high consumption of vegetables. Unhealthy fats are replaced with olive oil and other healthy fats, while meat is limited.

microvascular complication   A long-term complication of diabetes related to the small blood vessels of the body. The commonly recognized microvascular complications include retinopathy (eyes), nephropathy (kidneys), and neuropathy (nerves).

monounsaturated fatty acids (MUFAs)   Fat molecules that have only one double bond or unsaturated carbon. MUFAs can help lower LDL (bad) cholesterol and raise HDL (good) cholesterol.

motivation   An internal process that initiates, directs, and maintains behaviors. It can cause you to take action and to move toward a certain goal.

no-calorie sweetener   Also called *artificial sweetener, non-nutritive sweetener,* and *sugar substitute,* a highly intense sweetener used to sweeten foods without increasing calories.

obstructive sleep apnea (OSA)   A chronic condition that causes a temporary stoppage in breathing during sleep. Symptoms can include loud snoring with pauses and loud snorting or choking sounds when breathing starts again.

ophthalmologist   A medical doctor who specializes in the treating of eye disease.

optometrist   A doctor who provides primary eye and vision care.

osteoporosis   A condition of weak and brittle bones that increases the risk of bone fracture. Fractures due to bones weakened by osteoporosis are most likely to be in the hip, wrist, or spine.

overnutrition   A condition caused by eating too many low-nutrient, high-calorie foods and not getting enough activity. Inadequate vitamin, mineral, and fiber intake occurs even with a high volume of calories.

ovo-vegetarian   A vegetarian who eats eggs.

oxidation   A process by which a form of oxygen attaches to molecules, making them chemically unstable and resulting in cellular damage.

pancreas   A gland in the endocrine system that makes insulin.

pancreatitis   An inflammation of the pancreas, which can be acute or chronic.

peripheral neuropathy   A form of nerve damage that affects the nerves of the feet. Symptoms include pain, tingling, and numbness.

podiatrist   A doctor of podiatric medicine specializing in the diagnosis and treatment of foot and ankle conditions.

polycystic ovary syndrome (PCOS)   Occurs in women and teenage girls when reproductive hormones are out of balance. PCOS causes cysts to form on the ovaries and makes menstrual periods become infrequent or stop altogether. Acne and excess facial hair growth can also occur. PCOS is linked with insulin resistance and type 2 diabetes.

polypharmacy   A term used to describe multiple different prescription medications for various health conditions being taken at the same time.

polyunsaturated fatty acids (PUFAs)   Fat molecules that have more than one unsaturated carbon bond or double bond. PUFAs can help lower LDL (bad) cholesterol.

qualified health claim   A claim authorized by the FDA for nutrients that have supporting credible, scientific evidence they may be beneficial for a specific disease or health condition. For example, "calcium may reduce the risk of osteoporosis" is a qualified health claim because it's based on scientific studies.

registered dietitian   A food and nutrition expert who meets the requirements to qualify for the RD or RDN credential.

reservoir   The part of an insulin pump that holds the supply of insulin—usually the amount for two to three days.

resistance training   Also called *strength training,* exercise that causes the muscles to contract against an external resistance (which can be your own body weight, dumbbells, stretch bands, cans, or other items that cause your muscles to contract). This type of training improves strength, tone, the size of muscles, or endurance.

saturated fatty acids   Fat molecules that have no double bonds between the individual carbon atoms; the carbon atoms fully "saturated" with hydrogen atoms. Saturated fatty acids raise LDL (bad) cholesterol.

short-term diabetes complications   Blood glucose levels that go too low or too high and require urgent attention. Hypoglycemia is a short-term diabetes complication.

SMART   Refers to goals for behavior change that are specific, measurable, action-oriented, realistic, and timely.

subcutaneous injection   An injection into the layer of fat just under the surface of the skin.

systolic blood pressure   The upper number of a blood pressure reading, which represents when the heart contracts and pushes blood through the arteries.

triglycerides   A form of fat that is present in the blood and the body's fat stores. High triglycerides are a risk factor for heart disease.

type 1 diabetes   An autoimmune disease where the body's immune system destroys the cells in the pancreas that make insulin. People with type 1 diabetes must take insulin.

type 2 diabetes   A chronic condition that affects the way the body uses carbohydrates, which causes the blood glucose to go above normal.

vegan   Vegetarians who don't eat any animal products. They also don't use any products with animal-based ingredients. For example, many vegans avoid honey and don't use products made with wool, silk, or leather.

vegetarian   Someone who does not eat meat, fish, and poultry.

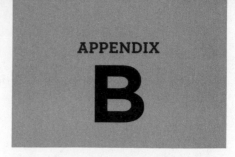

Resources for Diabetes Management

In this appendix, you'll find a number of diabetes management tools, including online resources, mobile applications, magazines, and books for tracking food, blood glucose, and activity. We hope you'll find these resources useful to help you successfully manage your diabetes.

Organization Resources

The following are official organizations that can help you get the correct facts on diabetes.

Academy of Nutrition and Dietetics
120 South Riverside Plaza, Suite 2000
Chicago, Illinois 60606
1-800-877-1600
eatright.org

The Academy of Nutrition and Dietetics is the world's largest organization of food and nutrition professionals. The Academy has over 75,000 members and is committed to improving the nation's health and advancing the profession of dietetics through research, education, and advocacy.

American Association of Diabetes Educators
200 West Madison Street, Suite 800
Chicago, IL 60606
1-800-338-3633
diabeteseducator.org

American Association of Diabetes Educators advocates on behalf of diabetes educators and the patients they serve. Their mission is to empower health-care professionals with the knowledge and skills to deliver exceptional diabetes education, management, and support.

American Diabetes Association
1701 North Beauregard Street
Alexandria, VA 22311
1-800-DIABETES (1-800-342-2383)
diabetes.org

The American Diabetes Association's mission is to prevent and cure diabetes and to improve the lives of all people affected by diabetes. The American Diabetes Association funds research to prevent, cure, and manage diabetes; delivers services to hundreds of communities; provides credible information; and advocates for people with diabetes.

National Diabetes Education Program
One Diabetes Way
Bethesda, MD 20814
301-496-3583
ndep.nih.gov

The National Diabetes Education Program is a federally funded program sponsored by the U.S. Department of Health and Human Services' National Institutes of Health and the Centers for Disease Control and Prevention. It includes over 200 partners at the federal, state, and local levels working together to improve the treatment and outcomes for people with diabetes, promote early diagnosis, and prevent or delay the onset of type 2 diabetes.

Online Resources

Navigating the internet to find credible resources can be a difficult task, so we've assembled some online resources on different areas associated with your health here.

Diabetes Education Programs

Programs recognized by the American Diabetes Association
professional.diabetes.org/erp_zip_search.aspx

Programs accredited by the American Association of Diabetes Educators
http://www.diabeteseducator.org/ProfessionalResources/accred/Programs.html

Exercise and Physical Activity

Activity tracker devices:

Fitbit
fitbit.com

Jawbone
jawbone.com

Vívofit
sites.garmin.com/en-US/vivo/vivofit/

Withings
withings.com

Modified physical activity:

Armchair Fitness
armchairfitness.com

Sit and Be Fit
sitandbefit.org

Nutrition and Meal Planning

The Center for Mindful Eating
thecenterformindfuleating.org/

Choose My Plate
choosemyplate.gov

Harvard School of Public Health (The Nutrition Source)
hsph.harvard.edu/nutritionsource

MyFoodAdvisor
tracker.diabetes.org

Oldways
oldwayspt.org

Physicians Committee for Responsible Medicine (Diabetes Resources)
pcrm.org/health/diabetes-resources

University of Georgia Cooperative Extension (Sample Menus)
spock.fcs.uga.edu/ext/pubs/food.php?category=Diabetes

Complementary and Alternative Medicine

Health Journeys
healthjourneys.com

National Center for Complementary and Integrative Health
nccih.nih.gov

National Institutes of Health Office of Dietary Supplements
ods.od.nih.gov

Quitting Smoking

The Centers for Disease Control and Prevention (Tips from Former Smokers)
cdc.gov/tips

Smokefree.gov
smokefree.gov

Weight Management

CalorieKing
calorieking.com

GoMeals
gomeals.com

Myfitnesspal
myfitnesspal.com

Nutrition.gov (Weight Management)
nutrition.gov/weight-management

SparkPeople
sparkpeople.com

Supertracker
supertracker.usda.gov

Parents and Children

Be Healthy Today, Be Healthy For Life: Information for Youth and Their Families Living with Type 2 Diabetes
http://main.diabetes.org/dorg/PDFs/Type-2-Diabetes-in-Youth/Type-2-Diabetes-in-Youth.pdf

Body Mass Index Percentile Calculator for Child and Teen
nccd.cdc.gov/dnpabmi/Calculator.aspx

Body Mass Index Percentile Chart for Girls Ages 2 to 20
cdc.gov/growthcharts/data/set2clinical/cj41l074.pdf

Body Mass Index Percentile Chart for Boys Ages 2 to 20
cdc.gov/growthcharts/data/set2clinical/cj41l073.pdf

ChooseMyPlate (MyPlate Kids' Place)
choosemyplate.gov/kids/

Ellyn Satter Institute
ellynsatterinstitute.org/index.php

Ibitz (pedometers)
ibitz.com

Safe at School
diabetes.org/living-with-diabetes/parents-and-kids/diabetes-care-at-school/

Older Adults

The Eldercare Locator
eldercare.gov

Go4Life (from the National Institute on Aging at NIH)
go4life.nia.nih.gov

Guide to Your Medicare Benefits
medicare.gov/publications/pubs/pdf/10116.pdf

National Diabetes Education Program (Diabetes Resources for Older Adults)
ndep.nih.gov/older-adults/

National Institute on Aging (Exercise)
nia.nih.gov/health/publication/exercise

Diabetes Magazines

These magazines offer information on living healthfully and managing your diabetes. Check out the websites for more information or to subscribe.

Diabetes Forecast
diabetesforecast.org/

Diabetes Self-Management
diabetesselfmanagement.com

Diabetic Living
diabeticlivingonline.com

Books on Diabetes

The following books give you information on things from fitness to meal planning when you have diabetes.

American Diabetes Association. *Month of Meals Diabetes Meal Planner.* Alexandria, VA: American Diabetes Association, 2010.

Geil, Patti B., and Tami A. Ross. *What Do I Eat Now?: A Step-by-Step Guide to Eating Right with Type 2 Diabetes, Second Edition.* Alexandria, VA: American Diabetes Association, 2015.

Hayes, Charlotte, MS. *The "I Hate to Exercise" Book for People with Diabetes: Turn Everyday Home Activities into a Low-Impact Fitness Plan You'll Love, Third Edition.* Alexandria, VA: American Diabetes Association, 2013.

Warshaw, Hope S., RD. *Diabetes Meal Planning Made Easy, Fourth Edition.* Alexandria, VA: American Diabetes Association, 2010.

———. *Eat Out, Eat Well.* Alexandria, VA: American Diabetes Association, 2015.

Record-Keeping Charts

In this appendix, we have provided some useful charts for you so you can record information that's important to manage your diabetes. Use these charts to keep track of the information not only for yourself, but also for your diabetes care team to review with them as needed. Feel free to make multiple copies of these for daily use, or go to idiotsguides.com/type2diabetes to print them out.

Diabetes Care Measures

The American Diabetes Association recommends certain treatment goals for good diabetes management, the measures of which are listed here. Use this chart at your doctor visits to track your diabetes measures.

Tests (How Often)	ADA Goal		My Goal	Date of Visit					
				Results					
A1C (Every 3–6 Months)	Below 7%								
Blood Pressure (Each Visit)	Below 140/90								
Cholesterol (Yearly)	Total	Below 200							
	LDL	Below 100							
	HDL	> 40 (Male)							
		> 50 (Female)							
Triglycerides (Yearly)	Below 150								
Foot Exam (Each Visit)									
Urine Test for Protein (Yearly)									
Blood Test for Kidney Function (GFR) (Yearly)									
Dilated Eye Exam (Yearly)									
Dental Exam (Every 6 Months)									
Flu Shot (Yearly)									
Weight (Each Visit)									

Check off (✓) the following when reviewed with your medical provider.

Blood Glucose (My Targets)	Before Meals: 80 to 130 mg/dL	Bedtime: 100 to 140 mg/dL				
Eating Well						
Exercise						
Blood Sugar Testing						
Blood Glucose Records						
High and Low Blood Sugar Frequency						
Medicine						
Daily Aspirin Use						
Foot Care						
Sick Day Care						
Stress Management						
Tobacco/Alcohol Use						

Date of Pneumonia Shot: _____

Completed Diabetes Self-Management Education Program: _____

Food and Blood Glucose Record

Use the following food and blood glucose record to keep track of your blood glucose results and food intake to help you identify if any changes are needed in your meal plan. You don't have to test your blood glucose before and after every meal, depending on what you are trying to find out. Talk with your medical provider about how often you should test your blood glucose.

Date	Before Time ---- Result	Breakfast	After Time ---- Result	Before Time ---- Result	Lunch	After Time ---- Result	Before Time ---- Result	Dinner	After Time ---- Result	Bedtime
	---		---	---		---	---		---	
	---		---	---		---	---		---	
	---		---	---		---	---		---	

Date	Before Time ---- Result	Breakfast	After Time ---- Result	Before Time ---- Result	Lunch	After Time ---- Result	Before Time ---- Result	Dinner	After Time ---- Result	Bedtime

Blood Glucose Record for Insulin Users

Use the following record to record the time your insulin dose was taken, along with what type and how many units in the section to the left. To the right, list the time you took your blood glucose and the result in the appropriate column.

Date	Insulin							Blood Glucose Results											
	Type	Dose					Test		Breakfast		Lunch		Dinner		Bedtime	Night	Notes
		Morning	Noon	Evening	Night				Before	2 Hours After	Before	2 Hours After	Before	2 Hours After			
						Time Taken	Time of Test										
							Blood Glucose										
						Time Taken	Time of Test										
							Blood Glucose										

Date	Insulin			Blood Glucose Results									
	Time Taken			Time of Test	Blood Glucose		Time of Test	Blood Glucose		Time of Test	Blood Glucose		Time of Test	Blood Glucose

Food Record Rating Hunger and Fullness

If you've become out of touch with your physical feelings of hunger and fullness, you can use this one-day record to improve your awareness by rating your hunger and fullness level before and after eating. Use the column to the right to record any observations about what type of foods you chose, size of portions, or emotions surrounding the eating episode. Copy this for a week's worth of records.

Time	Hunger Level Before Eating (0 to 5)	Foods	Hunger Level Before Eating (0 to 5)	Observations About Food Choices, Portions Eaten, and Emotions (Like Stress or Boredom)

Hunger level key: 0 = Not hungry at all, 5 = Uncomfortably full.

Physical Activity Tracker

The following chart will help you track your weekly physical activity to ensure you're staying on the right track.

WEEK BEGINNING: ___/___/___   Weekly Activity Goal: _____

Weekly Activity Plan:

_____

_____

_____

_____

MONDAY:

Activity Type:

❑ Walking   ❑ Jogging   ❑ Treadmill   ❑ Swimming

❑ Biking   ❑ Exercise Class ❑ Other _____

Aerobic Activity (check one box for each 10 minutes of aerobic activity completed): ❑ ❑ ❑ ❑ ❑ ❑ ❑ ❑ ❑ ❑

Intensity: ❑ Easy   ❑ Medium   ❑ Hard

Resistance or Strength Training Activity:

❑ Weight Machine   ❑ Free Weights   ❑ Resistance Bands

❑ Body Weight Resistance (Push-Ups, Pull-Ups, etc.)   ❑ Other _____

Notes:

_____

_____

_____

_____

TUESDAY:

Activity Type:

❑ Walking   ❑ Jogging   ❑ Treadmill   ❑ Swimming

❑ Biking   ❑ Exercise Class   ❑ Other _____

Aerobic Activity (check one box for each 10 minutes of aerobic activity completed): ❑ ❑ ❑ ❑ ❑
❑ ❑ ❑ ❑ ❑

Intensity: ❑ Easy   ❑ Medium   ❑ Hard

Resistance or Strength Training Activity:

❑ Weight Machine   ❑ Free Weights   ❑ Resistance Bands

❑ Body Weight Resistance (Push-Ups, Pull-Ups, etc.)   ❑ Other _____

Notes:

_____

_____

_____

_____

WEDNESDAY:

Activity Type:

❑ Walking   ❑ Jogging   ❑ Treadmill   ❑ Swimming

❑ Biking   ❑ Exercise Class   ❑ Other _____

Aerobic Activity (check one box for each 10 minutes of aerobic activity completed): ❑ ❑ ❑ ❑ ❑
❑ ❑ ❑ ❑ ❑

Intensity: ❑ Easy   ❑ Medium   ❑ Hard

Resistance or Strength Training Activity:

❑ Weight Machine   ❑ Free Weights   ❑ Resistance Bands

❑ Body Weight Resistance (Push-Ups, Pull-Ups, etc.)   ❑ Other _____

Notes:

_____

_____

_____

_____

THURSDAY:

Activity Type:

❑ Walking   ❑ Jogging   ❑ Treadmill   ❑ Swimming

❑ Biking   ❑ Exercise Class   ❑ Other _____

Aerobic Activity (check one box for each 10 minutes of aerobic activity completed): ❑ ❑ ❑ ❑ ❑ ❑ ❑ ❑ ❑ ❑

Intensity: ❑ Easy   ❑ Medium   ❑ Hard

Resistance or Strength Training Activity:

❑ Weight Machine   ❑ Free Weights   ❑ Resistance Bands

❑ Body Weight Resistance (Push-Ups, Pull-Ups, etc.)   ❑ Other _____

Notes:

_____

_____

_____

_____

FRIDAY:

Activity Type:

❑ Walking   ❑ Jogging   ❑ Treadmill   ❑ Swimming

❑ Biking   ❑ Exercise Class   ❑ Other _____

Aerobic Activity (check one box for each 10 minutes of aerobic activity completed): ❑ ❑ ❑ ❑ ❑ ❑ ❑ ❑ ❑ ❑

Intensity: ❑ Easy   ❑ Medium   ❑ Hard

Resistance or Strength Training Activity:

❑ Weight Machine   ❑ Free Weights   ❑ Resistance Bands

❑ Body Weight Resistance (Push-Ups, Pull-Ups, etc.)   ❑ Other _____

Notes:

_____

_____

_____

_____

SATURDAY:

Activity Type:

❑ Walking   ❑ Jogging   ❑ Treadmill   ❑ Swimming

❑ Biking   ❑ Exercise Class   ❑ Other _____

Aerobic Activity (check one box for each 10 minutes of aerobic activity completed): ❑ ❑ ❑ ❑ ❑
❑ ❑ ❑ ❑ ❑

Intensity: ❑ Easy   ❑ Medium   ❑ Hard

Resistance or Strength Training Activity:

❑ Weight Machine   ❑ Free Weights   ❑ Resistance Bands

❑ Body Weight Resistance (Push-Ups, Pull-Ups, etc.)   ❑ Other _____

Notes:

_____

_____

_____

_____

SUNDAY:

Activity Type:

❏ Walking   ❏ Jogging   ❏ Treadmill   ❏ Swimming

❏ Biking   ❏ Exercise Class   ❏ Other _____

Aerobic Activity (check one box for each 10 minutes of aerobic activity completed): ❏ ❏ ❏ ❏ ❏ ❏ ❏ ❏ ❏

Intensity: ❏ Easy   ❏ Medium   ❏ Hard

Resistance or Strength Training Activity:

❏ Weight Machine   ❏ Free Weights   ❏ Resistance Bands

❏ Body Weight Resistance (Push-Ups, Pull-Ups, etc.)   ❏ Other _____

Notes:

_____

_____

_____

_____

Your Weight Record

Use the columns to the left to record your weekly weight, including the date and a running total of pounds lost each week. Use the graph on the right to record changes in your weight. Your starting weight should be graphed at 0 (toward the bottom of the page). Each square across represents one week, and each row represents 1 pound (either gained or lost starting from 0 on the graph).

Name: _____

Target Weight: _____

Week	Date	Weight	Pounds Lost
1			
2			
3			
4			
5			
6			
7			
8			
9			
10			
11			
12			
13			
14			
15			
16			

Graph row labels (top to bottom): +14, +13, +12, +11, +10, +9, +8, +7, +6, +5, +4, +3, +2, +1, 0, -1

	-2	-3	-4	-5	-6	-7	-8	-9	-10	-11	-12	-13	-14	-15	-16	-17	-18	-19	-20	-21	-22	-23	-24	-25

Week	Date	Weight	Pounds Lost
17			
18			
19			
20			
21			
22			
23			
24			
25			

Your Diabetes Care Team

Use this chart to list the contact information for each of the members of your diabetes care team.

Health-Care Provider	Location	Phone Number	Notes

Your Medication List

The following chart will help you list all of your medications in one place. Take this list with you to appointments with your diabetes care team. Keeping your providers informed about what medications you're taking will help you avoid duplicate medications and minimize the risk for adverse reactions.

Name: _____   Medication Allergies: _____

Medication (Brand Name or Generic Name)	Dose (How Much You Take)	How Often You Take It	Reason for Taking the Medication	Who Prescribed the Medication

SMART Goal-Setting Worksheet

Use this worksheet to develop SMART goals to better manage your diabetes. It's a good idea to choose no more than two goals at the same time.

What Is a SMART Goal?

Specific: Specifically state what you want to accomplish.

Measurable: How much or how often?

Action-oriented: What steps you will take to achieve your goal.

Realistic: It should be a bit of a challenge but not too difficult.

Timely: When will it happen?

Sample Goal Statement:

"I want to improve my blood glucose control to feel better and have more energy."

Sample Action Steps Using SMART Goal Setting:

Activity goal: "I will walk at the park for 30 minutes, in the morning before work, on Monday, Wednesday, and Friday this week."

Meal-planning goal: "I will choose fruit for a snack in the afternoon instead of chips or candy three days this week."

Now put your plan into action. What is your goal? List why you chose that goal.

_____

_____

_____

_____

What steps will you take to reach your goal? Make them SMART.

_____

_____

_____

_____

Index

glucose toxicity, 63
hydration, 206-207
hyperglycemia, 63
   medical emergencies, 64-65
   treating, 63-64
hypoglycemia, 59
   medical emergencies, 62
   preventing, 59-60
   treating, 60-62
menstrual cycle, 287
post-meal, 248-249
pre-meal, 246-247
protein, 151-152
target, attaining, 58-59
targets, 246
testing, 134-136
blood glucose meters, 136, 140-141
   accuracy, 136-138
   blood sample size, 139
   cost, 138-139
   finger pricking, 139-140
blood glucose tests, 9, 38
   A1C, 9-10, 16, 142
   c-peptide, 16
   children, 277-278
   fasting blood glucose, 9-10, 16
   OGTT (oral glucose tolerance test), 9-10
   perceived exertion, 77
   prior food intake, 10
   talk, 77
blood pressure, 143
BMI (body mass index), 27-28
   BMI-for-age, 275-276
board-certified in advanced diabetes management (BC-ADM), 51
body mass index (BMI), 27-28
boiling meats, 204
borderline diabetes, 4
brand names
   AGIs (alpha-glucosidase inhibitors), 117
   DDP-4 inhibitors, 116
   GLP-1 agonists, 120
   meglitinides, 115
   metformin, 112
   SGLT2 inhibitors, 119
   sulfonylurea, 114
   thiazolidinediones (TZDs), 118
Bromocriptine, 128
broth, low-sodium, 158
bulgur, 211
butter, compared to margarine, 183-184
Bydureon, 120
Byetta, 120

C

c-peptide test, 16
calcium-rich foods, 154
Calorie Counter & Diet Tracker, 217
calories, Nutrition Facts label, 169, 172, 179
Canagliflozin, 119
Carb Master, 217
carbohydrates, 29-30, 150-151, 216
   counting, 217-223
   snacks, 158
   total, Nutrition Facts label, 173
care team, creating, 48-54
Centers for Disease Control and Prevention, 32
central nervous system, 226
CFRD (cystic fibrosis–related diabetes), 21-22
chair stands, 75
children
   away-from-home plans, 282-286
   BMI-for-age, 275-276
   controlling environment, 280-281
   physical activity, 282
   risk factors, 274-278
   type 2 diabetes, 5
cholesterol, 143-145
cholesterol-free label claims, 170
ChooseMyPlate.gov, 32
chromium supplements, 97
chronic, 21
chronic pancreatitis, 20-21
cinnamon supplements, 95-96
clpidigrel (Plavix), 93
co-workers, support, 55-56
Colesevelam, 128

continuous glucose monitoring (CGM) system, 141

CoQ10 supplements, 93

cortisol, 104

cost
    blood glucose meters, 138-139
    medication, 263

Coumadin (warfarin), 93

counselors, 53

cravings, controlling, 26

curry powder, 158

Cycloset, 128

cystic fibrosis, 21-22

cystic fibrosis–related diabetes (CFRD), 21-22

D

Daily Carb Premium, 217

dairy, 155

Dapagliflozin, 119

DDP-4 inhibiters, 115-116

DE (diabetes educator), 249

dementia, 259

dentists, 53

depression, 105
    elderly, 260-261

detemir, 124

Diabeta, 114

diabetes educators (DEs), 50-51, 249

Diabetes Prevention Program (DPP). *See* DPP (Diabetes Prevention Program)

diabetic foods, 26

diabetic ketoacidosis (DKA), 15

diabetic nephropathy, 66

diabetic retinopathy, 66

diagnosing type 2 diabetes, 9-10

diet, 150-158
    balanced, 155-156
    butter versus margarine, 183-184
    carbohydrates, 29-30, 150-151
    eating out, 164-166
    enhancements, 158-159
    fad diets, 238-239
    fats, 152-153, 178-179

    MUFAs, 181-183
    PUFAs, 182-183
    trimming unhealthy, 179-181

fiber, 208-209

food labels
    front-package, 168-171
    nutrition facts, 171-176
    sugar, 197, 199

grocery shopping, 160-164

healthy, 29-30, 38

hurried eating, 242-244

labels, 150
    sugar, 197-199

macronutrients, 150

meal plans, 150, 216-217, 246
    counting carbohydrates, 217-223
    low-carb diet, 226-227
    Mediterranean, 228-231
    plate method, 223-226
    post-meal blood glucose, 248-249
    pre-meal blood glucose, 246-247
    Vegetarian, 232-235

meal replacements, 243-244

mindful eating, 239-241

nutrition, 264-265
    elderly, 265-268

nutritionists, 51-52

portion control, 26, 156-158

processed, 216

protein, 151-152
    lean, 202-205

reducing sodium, 185-188

safety, 266

substitutions, 159-160
    meat, 234

sweeteners, 197-199
    low-calorie, 190-191
    no-calorie, 192-197

water, 205-208

whole grains, 210-212

dietary supplements, 91
    alpha-lipoic acid, 94-95
    chromium, 97
    cinnamon, 95-96

Glipizide, 114
GLP-1 agonists, 120-121
glucagon, 115-116
glucagon-like peptide-1 (GLP-1), 116
Glucatrol, 114
Glucatrol XL, 114
Glucophage, 112
Glucophage XR, 112
glucose, 150
    toxicity, 63
Glumetza, 112
gluten free label claims, 168
Glyburide, 114
glycemic index (GI), 221-223
glycogen, 72
Glynase, 114
Glyset, 117
goals
    setting, 41-43
    SMART, 41-42, 250
    weight loss, 249-253
golfing, 270
"good" cholesterol, 86
grains, 154-155, 210-212
grocery shopping, 160-164
guided imagery, 107-108

H

Harvard School of Public Health, 32
HDL (high-density lipoprotein) cholesterol, 86, 144
health claims, 171
Health Journeys, 108
healthy diet. *See* diet
heart rate, measuring, 75-77
hemoglobin, 142
herbs, salt-free blends, 159
HHS (hyperosmolor hyperglycemic state), 64
high-density lipoprotein (HDL) cholesterol, 86, 144
hormones
    glucagon-like peptide-1 (GLP-1), 116
    incretin, 115-116
    stress, 104

hurried eating, 242-244
hydration, 205, 267
    blood glucose, 206-207
hydrogenated starch hydrolysates, 190
hyperglycemia, 4, 58, 63
    medical emergencies, 64-65
    treating, 63-64
hyperosmolor hyperglycemic state (HHS), 64
hypoglycemia, 58-59
    geriatrics, 259-260
    medical emergencies, 62
    preventing, 59-60
    treating, 60-62
    unawareness, 58

I

incretin, 115-116
inhaled insulin, 127-128
injuries, avoiding while exercising, 78-79
insoluble fiber, 208
insulin, 4, 122
    action times, 123
    administering, 125-128
    basal, 123-124
    inhaled, 127-128
    resistance, 4, 72
    supplementing, 6
insulin pumps, 128-131
intensity, physical exercise, 75-77
interstitial fluid, 141
Invokana, 119

J-K

Januvia, 116
Jardience, 119
Juvenile Diabetes Research Foundation, 31

kidney disease, 66
Klinefelter syndrome, 20

L

M

sodium free label claims, 170

sodium-glucose cotransporter 2 (SGLT2) inhibitors, 119

soluble fiber, 208

starches, 150

Starlix, 115

stevia, 195

strength training, 73-74, 270

 chair stands, 75

 wall push-ups, 74-75

stress, 103-104

 blood sugar effects, 104-105

 management, 105-107

 managing, 107-109

stress reduction resources, 43

substitutes

 meat, 234

 recipes, 196-197

substitutions, recipes, 159-160

sucralose, 195-196

sugar alcohols, 190-191

 side effects, 191

sugar consumption, 27

sugar free label claims, 170

sulfonylureas, 114

 side effects in elderly, 264

Supertracker, 44

supplements, 216

 proper use, 97-98

sustainable changes, making, 40-41

sweeteners, 197-199

 low-calorie, 190-191

 no-calorie, 192-197

swimming, 270

Symlin, 122

symptoms

 chronic pancreatitis, 21

 type 1 diabetes, 15

 type 2 diabetes, 8-9

syringes, 125-126

systolic blood pressure, 143

T

table salt compared to sea salt, 185

tai-chi, 109

talk test, 77

Tanzeum, 120-121

target blood glucose, attaining, 58-59

tempeh, 234

tenderizing meats, 205

tests, 38, 134-136

 A1C, 9-10, 16

 c-peptide, 16

 children, 277-278

 fasting blood glucose test, 9-10, 16

 OGTT (oral glucose tolerance test), 9-10

 perceived exertion, 77

 prior food intake, 10

 talk, 77

textured vegetable protein (TVP), 234

thiazolidinediones (TZDs), 118

tobacco smoking, 87-88

 benefits of not, 88

 weight gain after quitting, 89-90

 withdrawal, 89

tofu, 234

total carbohydrates, Nutrition Facts label, 173

Tradjenta, 116

trans fat free label claims, 170

trans fats, 180-181

treatments

 hyperglycemia, 63-64

 hypoglycemia, 60-62

 type 2 diabetes, 10

triglycerides, 144

Trulicity, 120-121

Turner syndrome, 20

TVP (textured vegetable protein), 234

type 1 diabetes, 6, 14

 causes, 14-15

 compared to type 2, 16

 demographics, 14